'Put yourself in my place'

Designing and managing care homes for people with dementia

Caroline Cantley and Robert C. Wilson

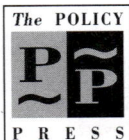

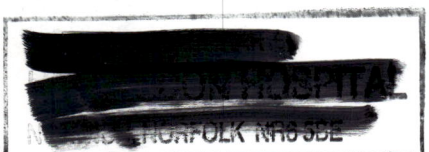

First published in Great Britain in March 2002 by

The Policy Press
34 Tyndall's Park Road
Bristol BS8 1PY
UK

Tel no +44 (0)117 954 6800
Fax no +44 (0)117 973 7308
E-mail tpp@bristol.ac.uk
www.policypress.org.uk

© The Policy Press 2002

In association with the Joseph Rowntree Foundation

ISBN 1 86134 389 2

Caroline Cantley is Professor of Dementia Care, University of Northumbria and Director, Dementia North and
Robert C. Wilson is a chartered civil engineer and a consultant offering specialised services in designing and building for care.

All rights reserved: no part of this publication may be reproduced, stored in a retrieval system, or transmitted in any form or by any means, electronic, mechanical, photocopying, recording or otherwise without the prior written permission of the Publishers.

The **Joseph Rowntree Foundation** has supported this project as part of its programme of research and innovative development projects, which it hopes will be of value to policy makers, practitioners and service users. The facts presented and views expressed in this report are, however, those of the authors and not necessarily those of the Foundation.

The statements and opinions contained within this publication are solely those of the authors and contributors and not of The University of Bristol or The Policy Press. The University of Bristol and The Policy Press disclaim responsibility for any injury to persons or property resulting from any material published in this publication.

The Policy Press works to counter discrimination on grounds of gender, race, disability, age and sexuality.

Cover design by Qube Design Associates, Bristol
Photograph on front cover supplied by the authors
Printed in Great Britain by Hobbs the Printers Ltd, Southampton

Contents

Acknowledgements	v
Preface	vii

Section One: Managing dementia care homes — 1

1 First steps in planning and establishing a dementia care home — 3
Introduction	3
Early planning	3
Establishing values and principles	4
Providing what people with dementia and their relatives want	5
Deciding on a service model	7
Deciding on the resident group	10
Providing for residents with specific needs	11
Opening the home	12

2 Management matters — 14
Introduction	14
Values and principles in practice	14
Management structures	14
Care home managers	16
Quality management	18
Staff management	20
Involving residents and relatives in management	22
Managing links with external services	22
Management development	24

3 Care matters — 25
Introduction	25
Person-centred care	25
Care planning	27
Therapies and activities	29
Mealtimes and nutrition	31
Physical and mental health	31
Managing medication	32
Palliative care, death and dying	32
Working with relatives	32
Community links	34
Residents' money	34
Risk management	34
Abuse	35
Legal and ethical issues	35

4 Staffing matters — 36
- Introduction — 36
- Staffing levels and skill mix — 36
- Staff recruitment — 39
- Staff induction — 40
- Staff retention — 41
- Staff work satisfaction — 41
- Pay and conditions of service — 42
- Staff development — 44

Section Two: Designing dementia care homes — 47

5 Design principles and processes — 49
- Introduction — 49
- Principles and features of good design — 49
- The design brief — 50
- Procurement methods — 51
- Managing the project — 52
- The design process: key messages — 52

6 Design in practice — 53
- Introduction — 53
- Home A — 53
- Home B — 56
- Home C — 62
- Home D — 66
- Home E — 71
- Home F — 75
- Home G — 80
- Learning from practice: key messages — 80

7 Design consensus and debates — 81
- Introduction — 81
- Consensus about 'best practice' — 81
- Debates about 'best practice' — 83
- Use of technology — 85

8 Design recommendations — 87
- Introduction — 87
- Size — 87
- Location — 88
- Design concept — 88
- Living areas — 88
- Service areas — 91
- Furniture and furnishings — 92
- Technology — 92
- Gardens and grounds — 92

9 Conclusion — 93

End notes — 94
Appendix: Comparison of various aspects of care homes visited — 108

Acknowledgements

We are grateful to the Joseph Rowntree Foundation who commissioned and funded this project. In particular we would like to thank Julie Cowans who initiated the project and Chrysa Apps who saw it through to completion. We are also indebted to members of the project Advisory Group for their support and comments throughout the work and to Loraine Barwick for taking and promptly circulating minutes. The names of the organisations that participated in the project are listed. During our case study visits, we met a very wide range of people from these organisations: senior managers, home managers, care staff and support staff. We also met architects and planners, staff and managers from some local health and social services agencies and, very importantly, people with dementia and their relatives. Everyone gave generously of their time, knowledge and experience; home managers especially were enormously helpful in organising our visits. Our thanks go to all of the above; to Tricia Leonard, Pat Harrison and Alwyne Wilson for help in preparation of the manuscript; to Orchard Print Services Ltd for producing the floor plans, and to the many unnamed others who helped to make this project possible.

Joseph Rowntree Foundation Advisory Group

Chrysa Apps, Practice Development Manager, Joseph Rowntree Foundation

Michael Broughton, Dementia Care Manager, Methodist Homes for the Aged

Wendy Bundy, Vice Chair, Selby and York Primary Care Trust

Julie Cowans, Housing Research Development Manager, Joseph Rowntree Housing Trust

J.C. Dennis, Director of Care Services, Joseph Rowntree Housing Trust

Valerie Good Anchor Housing Trust

Wendy Hatton, Regional Development Officer, Relatives Association

Dr Christine A. Kirk, Consultant Psychiatrist for the Elderly, York Health Services NHS Trust

John McNeil, McNeil & Beechey, Architects

Susan Mangeolles, Registration Officer, Bradford Social Services

Alex O'Neil, Research Manager, Joseph Rowntree Foundation

Tom Roche, Services Development Manager, The Retreat

Cilla Taggart, Manor House Nursing Home

Organisations involved in the study

The ExtraCare Charitable Trust

Humberside Independent Care Association Limited

Methodist Homes for the Aged

Orbit Housing Association

Quantum Care

Southern Cross Health Care

St John's Winchester Charity

Architects

ADW Partnership, Leicester

DBS, Nottingham

HSD Architects, Rickmansworth

PRP Architects, East Molesey

Rees Associates, Bury St Edmunds

Weaver Building Design, Bromsgrove

Design and build contractor

Castleoak Construction Healthcare, Newport

Preface

Introduction

Many people with dementia, if they have good support, can live out their lives in their own homes. However, for a significant number of people with dementia the support of a care home is the best option. As our understanding of the experience of dementia has advanced in recent years, so too has our understanding of how to improve the quality of life of people with dementia in care homes. One option is to develop specialist dementia care homes. However, care home providers who want to do this often find it difficult to obtain advice about what is involved in designing, setting up and maintaining a 'gold standard' dementia care home. This report aims to address the needs of care home providers. It draws on the experiences of seven specialist homes to advise on how to create and maintain a good place for people with dementia to live.

Service context

It is widely recognised that this is a challenging time for care home providers. First, care homes are responding to a wide range of policy and legislative[1] developments including:

- the introduction of the new regional Commissions for Care Standards
- the introduction of the single care home concept to replace nursing and residential home registration categories
- the introduction of national minimum standards
- the free provision of nursing care in homes
- changing requirements for staff training
- the establishment of the General Social Care Council to regulate social care personnel
- a growing policy emphasis on person-centred services
- the introduction of the 1998 Human Rights Act.

Second, care homes are responding to a range of economic pressures. Demand is depressed, local authority fees are not always keeping pace with cost increases and some homes, particularly small homes, are experiencing financial difficulties[2]. Homes are also coping with the implications of high employment rates and the introduction of the National Minimum Wage and the Working Time Directive. Such economic pressures, in combination with policy developments, have been leading to structural changes in the sector with a trend towards larger homes and increasing corporatisation[3].

Third, care homes are adapting to significant changes in their resident populations. They increasingly provide services for the very oldest people who have multiple and complex needs. Consequently, they are providing care for growing numbers of people with dementia. In England, there are approximately 46,500 places designated for people aged 65 years and over with mental health problems; approximately 23,000 in residential homes and approximately 23,500 in private nursing homes, hospitals and clinics[4]. However, these figures substantially underestimate the numbers involved as various studies have found that between 30% and almost 80%[5] of residents in residential homes have dementia; this means that we can expect to find between around 72,000 and 192,000 people with dementia in residential homes in England[6]. Alzheimer's Scotland Action on Dementia provides similar detailed estimates for Scotland[7]. These very substantial numbers of people with dementia in care homes are creating demands on managers and staff that provider organisations must address[8].

The National Service Framework for Older People[9] recommends that the National Health Service, local authorities and independent care providers should work together to develop specialist dementia care places. This will give many provider organisations an added impetus to consider the development of specialist dementia care homes or units within homes. Providers embarking on this type of development have two main concerns: improving the quality of their services and maintaining the financial viability of their businesses. In producing this guide we are very aware that care home providers must operate 'in the real world' and that different providers have to cope with different constraints. We have, therefore, based this guidance on a range of case studies. In so doing we aim to show how much can be achieved when providers have the will to translate the principles of good dementia care into the reality of everyday life in a care home.

Our case studies

This report is based on seven case studies and a literature review. We started from the view that the character and quality of a care home is shaped by the building, the provider organisation and the residents[10]. We were also mindful of the importance of taking into account the different interests and concerns of different groups including residents, relatives, staff, home managers, and staff in related services.

In selecting the case study homes, we aimed to obtain a very broad picture of different types of specialist dementia care home. Our 'sample' was based on the following requirements:

- each home should provide specialist dementia care either throughout or in substantial dedicated sections
- each home should be in a new building, designed specifically for people with dementia and in use long enough for staff to have 'evaluated' it
- each home and/or organisation should be recommended by 'experts' in the field as having a reputation for good dementia care
- there should be a mix of different types of parent provider organisation
- there should be a mix of homes of different sizes and structures.

Each case study visit took place over two days and was sometimes supplemented by an additional visit or interviews. The visits generally involved:

- detailed individual interviews with managers and other staff
- interviews with architects and other building professionals
- group interviews with care staff
- group interviews and discussions with relatives
- informal discussions with staff, relatives and residents
- informal observation of the day-to-day life in the home
- a 'tour' of the building and gardens
- a structured survey of the environment.

We also occasionally had opportunities to observe staff meetings, residents' meetings and meetings of relatives' groups. Although we had some informal conversations with people with dementia living in the homes, we were not able to involve them in the project as much as we would have liked. It is clear that people with dementia in care homes can express views about their lives[11]. However, the techniques that we would have wanted to use to hear their views would have required a time commitment that was beyond the scope of this project.

In order to preserve confidentiality, we have not named individual homes or respondents in this guide.

The homes in the study

Table 1 shows how the seven case study homes varied in type, size, basic structure and parent provider organisation.

Preface

Table 1: Case study homes

Home	Category	Size	Structure of units	Additional services	Parent provider organisation
A	Nursing	36	4 dementia units x 9 beds		Charity
B	Residential	36	3 dementia units x 12 beds		Charity
C	Residential	60	1 dementia unit x 15 beds; 3 units x 15 beds for physically frail older people	10 place day centre operating 6 days/week Respite care for day care clients – no dedicated respite places	Not for profit
D	Dual registered	24	3 dementia units x 8 beds	1 bed used for respite	Housing association
E	Residential	72	2 dementia units x 24 beds; 1 unit x 24 beds for physically frail older people	Occasional respite – no dedicated respite places	Not for profit
F	Nursing	23	2 dementia units x 8 beds; 1 dementia unit x 7 beds	10 place day centre operating 3 days/week 3 x respite beds in separate unit	Charity
G	Nursing	60	1 dementia unit x 30 beds; 1 unit x 30 beds for physically frail older people	Occasional respite – no dedicated respite places	Private

Using this guide

This guide has two sections. Section One deals with the planning, management, practice and staffing issues that are essential components of creating high quality living environments for people with dementia. This section will be of interest to two main groups: senior managers who are considering, or embarking on the development of a specialist dementia care home; and, the managers of both new and established dementia care homes. Section Two deals with planning, designing, building and maintaining the type of physical environments that are important for the quality of life of people with dementia. This section will be of interest to planners, architects, project managers and other senior managers involved in property development. It will also be useful for managers of new and existing homes who have opportunities to influence interior design and fittings.

Section One:
Managing dementia care homes

First steps in planning and establishing a dementia care home

Introduction

This chapter addresses the issues that provider organisations face in the early stages of setting up dementia care homes. It begins with some advice about service planning. It then discusses values and principles; providing what people with dementia and their relatives want; service models; deciding on the nature of the resident group; and providing for residents with specific needs. It ends with advice about how to achieve success in the opening stages of a new home.

Early planning

Specialist homes for people with dementia are set up in different circumstances, for different reasons, by different provider organisations with different prior experiences of care home provision and of dementia care. In our study, for example, homes variously had their origins in:

- reprovision of longstay NHS hospital beds
- replacement of former local authority homes by transfer to the independent sector
- speculative development based on market analysis.

A provider's decision to set up a specialist dementia care home may be, for example:

- part of a strategy for developing specialist dementia care homes within a broader and expanding portfolio of services
- part of a strategy to reconfigure existing services to meet local market needs more effectively and efficiently
- an opportunistic move into a new area of provision
- a new organisation's first service venture.

Because of the above differences, the process of setting up a new home may involve:

- designing, building and opening a new home 'from scratch'
- decanting residents and staff from an existing home and moving them back some months later into a new building
- bringing together in a new building staff and residents from other homes that have been closed
- relocating to a new building the 'patients' and staff from former NHS hospital wards.

Since homes originate in different circumstances, the experience of and feelings involved in opening a new home vary. For most organisations, there is the excitement and challenge of development and change. However, if the development is driven by financial and property pressures, this enthusiasm may be tempered by having to deal with some difficult political, resource and personnel constraints.

Although different providers embarking on the development of a dementia care home have different experiences, they also face many similar challenges. Based on our case studies, we summarise some broad ranging advice for providers as they take the first steps to establish a specialist dementia care home (see Box 1.1). We deal with many of these points in greater detail in later sections of this report.

Box 1.1: Planning dementia care homes: first steps

- Set out with a commitment to achieve best practice in dementia care.
- Do not underestimate the scale and difficulty of the task of setting up a new home.
- Ensure values and principles are explicit and shape the initiative from the outset.
- Ensure that plans take full account of what people with dementia and relatives want.
- Discuss plans with registration and inspection authorities from an early stage in the process.
- Discuss plans with service commissioners and potential purchasers from an early stage in the process to establish the basis of demand, contracting, fees, quality requirements and so on.
- Develop a clear service model from an early stage.
- Decide who the home will provide for and what services it will provide.
- Consider the location of the home very carefully. Which local authorities will be purchasers? How will residents and families perceive the location? How will the location affect access for staff and families?
- Ensure good building design (see Section Two) but do not let the demands of getting a good building dominate over other issues.
- Establish good community links from the planning stages. There may be a need to overcome resistance to the home from local communities who think its location undesirable.
- Develop, from the outset, good partnership working with other local services. For example, other services may need convincing that the home will have the necessary expertise to care for people with dementia; and, GPs in particular may view the home as an unwelcome additional demand on their time.
- Be alert to any changes in the environment that may affect the setting up or operation of the home. For example, organisational, personnel or financial changes in other agencies may affect their purchasing of places or ability to provide support services.
- Do not underestimate the importance of getting the best managers and staff. As one manager commented, "design is part of it and concept is part of it but at the end of the day people are crucial". Assess the employment market and plan accordingly.
- Invest time in recruiting the best possible home manager.
- Ensure the manager is appointed or designated well before the home opens (in study homes the shortest period was six weeks but the recommended period was up to eight months).
- Involve the manager as soon as possible in building work, ideally to comment on design but at least to comment on the details of internal fittings.
- Involve the manager as soon as possible in decisions about staffing issues and management systems.

Establishing values and principles

One of the essential tasks in setting up a new dementia unit is establishing clear values and principles for the service. Values and principles are in part home-specific and dementia-specific but they also, to varying extents, reflect the values and philosophies of parent provider organisations.

Homes for people with dementia should operate in accord with the accepted values and principles for care homes more generally[12]. Additionally, value statements for dementia care, such as that produced by the King's Fund[13], particularly emphasise the unique human existence of each person with dementia and the interdependency between them and other people. Another framework describes the following five core values for dementia care services:

- maximising personal control
- enabling choice
- respecting dignity
- preserving continuity (of lived experience and care provision)
- promoting equity[14].

Organisations can use this framework to interpret the values in their particular service context and to monitor provision against their values.

Although good dementia care homes must share the same broad set of values and principles there may be differences in emphasis. For example, two of our study homes placed particular emphasis on Christian values and one emphasised

> **Box 1.2: Some important values and principles in dementia care homes**
>
> - Respecting residents' rights
> - Ensuring residents' privacy and dignity
> - Tailoring care to individual and changing needs
> - 'Knowing the person'
> - Maximising abilities and independence
> - Recognising the importance of relatives and friends
> - Managing risk appropriately
> - Promoting choice
> - Empowering residents, relatives and staff
> - Valuing and trusting staff
> - Open-mindedness
> - Honesty
> - Love
> - Homeliness
> - Friendliness
> - Calmness and peacefulness
> - Harmony
> - Trust

family values. The important values and principles shared by the homes in this study are summarised in Box 1.2. Homes express their values and principles in a variety of ways including mission statements, value statements and residents' charters.

Providing what people with dementia and their relatives want

It is increasingly accepted that care homes need to take much greater account of the views and preferences of the people who live there, including people with dementia. Research on what people with dementia want from services is expanding[15] but there is as yet relatively little that sheds light on what is important to people with dementia in care homes. We know more about what older people in general want from care homes. The priorities of people with dementia may well be different from those of the wider population of older residents. However, given the lack of specific research on this count, it is reasonable to take the views of older people in general as a starting point and to assume that for people with dementia we need at least to meet, and no doubt in some respects to exceed, these general expectations.

A number of studies shed light on the things that are important to older people in care homes[16]. The social factors that are important include:

- recreational activities
- social relationships with like-minded people
- good company and friendship of other residents
- visitors
- opportunities to get out (including availability of transport)
- spiritual aspects, including maintaining religious contacts
- good atmosphere based on friendly, respectful relationships between residents and between residents and staff.

The regime and care provided are also important and specific factors include:

- maintenance of individuality and a sense of self
- choice (particularly in personal routines)
- meals and food (including having a choice of food and opportunities to make drinks)
- care from kind and knowledgeable staff
- continuity of staffing
- support service availability
- personal safety
- aids and adaptations to promote self-care
- privacy
- ability to come and go at will
- staff using preferred manner of address
- choice of gender of staff for intimate care
- control over money.

And, the environment of the home is important. Significant factors identified in the literature include:

- physical comfort and amenities (including en suite toilets)
- furniture (including having own furniture brought in)
- access to own bedroom at any time (including the facility to eat in own room)
- the size of the home
- locks on bedroom doors
- two sitting areas – one a quiet lounge.

Relatives

From discussions with relatives during our case study visits, we identified the aspects of the home that were important to them (see Box 1.3). The factors identified by relatives as being important are on very many counts similar to the factors that from the literature we identified above as being important for residents[17].

Box 1.3: Relatives' views about what is important in a dementia care home

Good care for the person with dementia, including:
- dignity, privacy and respect for the person with dementia
- individuality in care
- making the person with dementia feel special (for example through affectionate physical touch such as hand holding or a kiss)
- clothes carefully laundered and returned to rightful owner
- ensuring that the person is always clean and well dressed
- appropriate activity and stimulation
- plenty of outings
- good meals.

A good physical environment, including:
- security in the home
- a pleasant, homely environment
- plenty of space in the home
- a nice garden
- design appropriate for people with dementia
- good location in the community
- having somewhere in the home semi-private and comfortable to see the resident other than in the resident's own room
- geographical accessibility by private and public transport
- pleasant, clean and comfortable environment
- no unpleasant odours.

A good social environment, including:
- homely, family atmosphere ("one big family", "it's like coming home")
- loving atmosphere ("there's an abundance of love in this building, it's patently obvious, it's there, you can see it")
- happy atmosphere ("my mother is laughing and smiling in this home and that's something to be grateful for")
- people not "sitting around the walls".

Good staff whose qualities include:
- skill
- kindness and caring.

A good response to relatives, including:
- easy relaxed relationships between relatives and staff
- relatives being made to feel welcome
- relatives feeling able to influence care ("you can just say, they take notice and don't take offence")
- contact with and support from other relatives
- appreciation of relatives and their feelings ("we, as relatives, are valued, cared about; we are part of this place. If [the residents] are so well looked after we don't feel so guilty, so bad").

Deciding on a service model

A key question for providers considering a specialist dementia facility is the extent to which dementia care is different from care provision for older people more generally. Several managers in this study argued that there are few fundamental differences in managing specialist dementia care homes or units. Our study homes, however, had dementia-specific features in many areas such as:

- environmental design
- size of units and staff:resident ratios
- management expertise
- provision of therapies and activities
- risk management
- staff training.

Homes vary in the extent to which they explicitly link their service model to theory and research in dementia care. None of our study homes used a model of dementia care that we could identify as being in all respects superior to other approaches. The words of one manager sum this up: "It is about core values expressed through a variety of models". Indeed, managers talked about the importance of having different service configurations in homes and different cultures or atmospheres in order to offer people choice. For example, one manager acknowledged that her home was friendly, with lots of joking and humour and quite a lot of noise. While she saw this as being part of the home's strengths, she recognised that it would not be everyone's choice.

Which model of care?

The separate registration of nursing and residential homes will cease in April 2002 with the introduction of the single care home concept[18]. However, debates are likely to continue well beyond this about whether nursing models or social care models are more appropriate in dementia care homes. In making decisions about the model of care to be adopted, it is important to be clear about the factors involved. For example, a home may make the case for having a nursing model purely on the grounds of care benefits or it may also be influenced by economic factors such as the higher fees and better staff:resident ratios that accompany nursing care.

The study homes that advocated a nursing lead generally argued that since dementia is 'a major illness' it is important to have RMN (Registered Mental Nurse) trained nursing staff to undertake assessments, to deal with residents with challenging behaviour and to work with relatives. The case was often made for also having trained RGNs (Registered General Nurses) to deal with physical problems. There is some evidence that when homes have nursing staff, the residents have better levels of orientation but also higher levels of apathy (possibly attributable to nurses' expectation of 'patients')[19]. Homes adopting a nursing-led model certainly need to consider social models of care if they are to ensure that medical and task-oriented nursing approaches do not preclude more holistic approaches and the social benefits that people with dementia can derive from residential care facilities[20].

The study homes that advocated a social care model generally argued that the needs of people with dementia are best met in an environment that is as ordinary as possible and that a social care model is better suited to providing this than a nursing model. They considered it perfectly possible to meet the healthcare needs of people with dementia in care homes without having a nursing lead or qualified nursing staff.

Of course nursing and social care are not necessarily mutually exclusive alternatives. In practice, good homes incorporate the best elements of both models. Moreover, there are other variants. For example, one home in our study was set up by a housing association and had a strong emphasis in the planning stages on what it called 'a housing rather than medical model'. This model drew heavily on social models of care but with a particularly strong emphasis on the building being 'the residents' home'.

Managers in all of our homes used this notion of the 'residents' home' to contrast their service with hotel, hospital or other institutional services. However, there were differences between the homes in how the notion of 'the residents' home' was translated into practice and some homes recognised their limitations in achieving this ideal:

"I don't think residential care can ever be home no matter how hard we try."
(Manager)

A home for life?

Providing a 'home for life' is a commonly held goal in dementia care in this country, although practice in other countries suggests that we should not accept this unquestioningly as being the best option in all circumstances[21]. Home managers in our study all espoused the view that since 'this is the resident's home' it is as far as possible their 'home for life'. Moreover, all of the managers claimed success in achieving this goal. This was as true of residential homes as nursing homes. Managers and staff in residential homes explained that with appropriate support from general and psychiatric community nursing services, they could meet the needs of all residents with dementia apart from those requiring acute hospital treatment.

A specialist home or integrated specialist units?

There can be problems in settings in which people with dementia live alongside other 'non-confused' residents[22]. One suggestion, to avoid adverse effects on the quality of life for both groups of residents and to avoid undue burden on staff, is that the proportion of 'confused' residents should be controlled[23]. However, in determining the appropriate mix of residents we must take into account many other factors such as staffing levels and skills and the effect of structuring homes into specialist units. Overall, there is no definitive evidence about the relative merits of separate dementia homes compared with specialist dementia units. Nor is there definitive evidence about the best way to structure and manage specialist dementia units.

Providers who opt for specialist dementia units should consider the extent to which the units will be integrated and how the interaction between different staff and resident groups will be managed. At one end of the spectrum of integration, residents in the 'dementia unit' may be included fully in the general life of the home, for example by being free to spend time and perhaps to have meals in other units. At the other end of the spectrum, there may be very little contact at all between the staff and residents of 'dementia units' and those of other units. The homes in our study with dementia units highlighted a number of points about this issue of integration. The main advantages of well integrated specialist units are that people with dementia benefit from the stimulation and social contact provided by other residents and that it is less likely that there will be problems with people with dementia becoming agitated by being contained within one unit. However, integration must be handled carefully to avoid problems. The issues that may need to be addressed include: residents of the dementia unit being viewed negatively and being socially rejected by other residents; residents who do not have dementia complaining about the disruptive behaviour of some people with dementia; and some families of people who do not have dementia objecting to their relative 'being with people like that'.

How big a home and what size of units?

There is broad agreement that it is desirable for dementia care homes to be small scale.

'Small scale' may refer to the size of the home overall or to the size of units within a larger home[24]. There is little evidence about the optimal size of larger homes composed of small-scale units. In general a philosophy of 'ordinary living' and anti-institutionalisation points to keeping the overall size of the home as small as possible.

The advantages of small-scale units have been identified as follows[25]:

- people with dementia are not overloaded with stimuli of noise, activity and too many other people
- the design can be domestic and hence more familiar
- it is easier for people with dementia to participate in domestic activities
- it is easier for staff to get to know individual residents
- unit-based staff groups facilitate the development of the team spirit and expertise that produces good dementia care.

In our study homes, managers and staff favoured small-scale units. They often made this point by drawing comparison with their own experience of working in homes with larger units where they felt that the quality of care was much poorer.

Managers and staff identified the following advantages of small-scale units:

- people with dementia experience less stress in smaller units and do not 'set each other off' so much
- relatives are not 'swamped' when they visit and they are more likely to get to know other relatives
- it is easier to develop good resident–keyworker relationships
- it is easier for staff to be clear about which residents they are responsible for
- it is easier for staff to keep an eye on all residents
- staff develop a greater sense of ownership and pride in their unit.

However, the intensity of small-scale units may carry a greater risk of staff 'burn out'[25]. In addition, staffing flexibility in the home as a whole may be inhibited if staff are dedicated to individual units. All of our study homes tried as far as possible to maintain consistent staff groups on their units. However, one home (Home F), which had units with quite different dependency levels, adopted a system of six-monthly rotation of senior care staff and three-monthly rotation of qualified nurses and care staff. The manager suggested that this reduced staff stress levels, increased staff learning and had no adverse effects on residents.

Definitions of what constitutes 'small scale' in the context of dementia care units vary from six to around 14 residents[26]. Staff and managers in our study with experience of small units suggested ideal sizes ranging from six to 12 residents per unit. They suggested that as the size of the unit increases there is a move away from having a 'family feel' in the home. In general, the unit size favoured by staff in our homes was slightly smaller than that in their current home – as long as staffing was maintained at the existing level.

Unit sizes in our study homes were determined by an interplay of factors, including homes:

- having a desire to keep units as small as possible
- using multiples of the staff:resident ratio (sometimes with the compromise of having additional staff 'floating' between units)
- holding views about how staff teams best operate (for example, some homes favoured staff working in groups of three on a unit while others favoured staff working in pairs)
- matching unit size with building design ratios for bathrooms and toilets.

Two study homes (Homes E and G) had a unit size that substantially exceeded the size recommended above. The main reason for this was financial viability. While recognising the disadvantages of larger units, these organisations argued that management is more important than numbers in securing good quality care. Certainly, the size of a facility is only one of many factors influencing the quality of care[27]. However, no matter how high the quality of care provided, the experience of living and working in a large-scale facility is fundamentally different from that of smaller units.

Should units have different dependency levels?

In three of our four dedicated dementia care homes, there was no policy of differentiating need across units. The managers argued that it was pointless to do this as residents change at different rates and in different ways. The fourth home grouped residents in units according to level of dependency. The manager suggested that it was easier to provide good care on a unit when residents had similar levels of need. Moreover, since staff rotated between units they still gained experience of working with residents with different abilities and this helped them to maintain high expectations of what can be achieved with people with dementia.

Should the home provide short-term care or day care?

Combining long-term and short-term care in one setting can be difficult for short-term residents, can be disruptive for long-term residents and can create problems of conflicting demands for staff[28]. The homes in our study that provided respite or day care were aware of the potential problems but felt that they could minimise any difficulties and that any disadvantages were outweighed by the benefits of offering these services. They identified two main benefits of having respite and day care places: staff can get to know service users and relatives at an earlier stage; people with dementia can become familiar with the home before they reach the point of moving in as a permanent resident.

Providers who consider including respite or day care in their home must be clear about the type of service that will be offered and what it is aiming to achieve[29]. For example, does the service aim to provide:

- maintenance or improvements in the functioning of the person with dementia
- improved quality of life for the person with dementia
- regular breaks for carers to help them to keep someone with dementia at home
- direct support services for carers
- emergency care, for example, in cases of carer illness
- temporary placements until permanent arrangements can be made
- opportunities for people with dementia to get to know the home with a view to eventual placement?

Providers should also be clear about the range of needs that they can accommodate and the implications of having a mixed client group, for example of people with very different levels of dementia. The stance taken on all of the above will inform service configurations and staffing. From the literature[30] we can identify important features of respite and day care. These are very similar to the features of good care home provision that we are advocating. Thus, good respite and day care facilities will have:

- clarity of purpose
- provision on a small scale
- a homely, welcoming environment
- individualised care based on knowing the person with dementia
- good quality care including occupation and stimulation
- staff skilled and experienced in dementia care
- good communication between carers, staff and the person with dementia
- staff recognition of carers' knowledge and expertise
- staff able to work in partnership with carers
- flexibility in the availability of the service
- continuity of staff
- good links with other services
- accessibility
- good preparation of the person with dementia and carers prior to the stay.

Deciding on the resident group

Recent research has highlighted how affinity between residents is important in shaping the atmosphere and quality of life in care homes[31]. It is therefore important that providers consider the extent to which the home will have a homogeneous or mixed resident population in terms of dependency and other resident characteristics including: age, gender, social background, religious background, and cultural and ethnic origins. We consider below provision for two groups with specific needs: younger people with dementia and people from minority ethnic communities.

The levels of dependency in specialist dementia care homes and units vary considerably[32]. For example, two of our study homes (A and D) concentrated on residents with high levels of dependency who could not be cared for readily in other care homes. Some other study homes (for example C and E) provided for people with a very broad range of dependency levels. If homes are to control the overall dependency level of their resident population, they must be clear about their admission and discharge criteria. These criteria are determined by the provider's views about the levels of dependency and behavioural difficulty that can be handled in the home and by the extent to which there is a commitment to providing 'a home for life' (see page 8). The case for using standard measures to assist in the management of overall dependency levels has been well made[33]. Our study homes made limited use of standard measures and managers generally were cautious that such measures can all too easily become inappropriate 'dependency labels' for residents.

'New start' homes are likely to experience two trends in their resident population. First, the initial intake of residents may include few people whose dementia is severe because referring agencies are at that stage unsure of the ability of the home to cope. However, as the home becomes more established and demonstrates its ability to provide high quality care, referrers begin to seek admission for people who present a greater challenge. Second, the residents who are admitted initially become more dependent as their dementia progresses. Both trends mean that new homes have to keep staffing ratios and rotas under review to cope with changing needs.

Providing for residents with specific needs

Younger people with dementia

It is only recently that the particular needs of people with early onset dementia have come to the fore[34]. A particular problem for this group is the limited availability of specialist residential accommodation. Younger people with dementia who need long-term care are often admitted to homes for older people and three of our homes had experience of providing care for younger residents. The managers felt that a home geared to older people was not ideal for these younger residents, but that in practice the arrangements had worked reasonably well. There is as yet limited research-based advice available for organisations on how the specific needs of younger people with dementia are best met in residential settings.

Residents from minority ethnic and cultural communities

Similarly, we have only recently begun to recognise the needs of people with dementia from minority ethnic communities[35]. It is important to stress that as well as paying attention to people from black and Asian communities we must pay attention to the needs of other groups who may be culturally, linguistically, spiritually or socially disadvantaged in care homes (for example, people who are Jewish or whose origins were in Eastern Europe). Anecdotally we know that some people from minority ethnic or cultural communities end up in mainstream provision that does not have the expertise to provide appropriate care[36]. There are arguments for homes to be developed for people from specific minority ethnic or cultural communities. However, we limit ourselves here to commenting on how needs may best be met in homes that include people from a mix of ethnic and cultural backgrounds.

Our study homes had very limited experience of providing care for residents from minority ethnic or cultural groups and there is little other available research. However, drawing on some earlier and broader work[37], we identify in Box 1.4 some basic advice for homes considering the provision of care for residents with dementia from minority ethnic or cultural communities.

Box 1.4: Providing care for residents with dementia from minority ethnic and cultural communities

- Do not make stereotypical assumptions about people based on their ethnic or cultural backgrounds; recognise the diversity that exists within communities and respond accordingly.
- Be clear about the minority ethnic and cultural groups for which the service is to be provided.
- Ensure that the perspectives of the relevant communities are addressed in all policies and practices.
- Ensure that staff can communicate with residents and their families in ways and in languages that are appropriate.
- Person-centred care must be ethnically and culturally appropriate, so homes should:
  - respond appropriately to any particular physical needs of the residents, relating, for example, to diet, health, skin care;
  - ensure that the residents' social needs are addressed including appropriate occupation and leisure activities, and maintenance of family and community links;
  - use 'life story' work to develop the staff's understanding of the ethnic and cultural background of the resident;
  - respect residents' spiritual backgrounds and make the necessary arrangements for them to fulfil the practices of their faith.
- Ensure that the staff group includes people who know and understand the past social world of the resident and the implications of the past for current needs; ideally there should be staff who share the ethnic and cultural background of residents.
- Ensure that staff supervision addresses racism and broader race and cultural issues.
- Develop good links with key people and organisations within the relevant ethnic and cultural communities.

Opening the home

Setting up a home and moving into a new building is a major project that taxes management skills to the full. Managers in our homes identified a wide range of practical arrangements as being important for a successful start. Based on their comments, we summarise general advice about 'opening a home' in Box 1.5. Advice that is more specifically related to new homes that involve relocation of residents is contained in Box 1.6.

Relocation raises questions about the possible adverse effects for people with dementia. Since relocation is sometimes linked with increased mortality, it is wise to act to ensure that disruption is minimised. Important action points are summarised below based on the recommendation of a recent review[38] and on our case studies:

- Assess the risks of transfer for each individual.
- Plan the move carefully and in detail.
- Monitor the process of the move carefully.
- Ensure the appropriate involvement of GPs and other clinicians.
- Maintain existing keyworker relationships where possible and appropriate; decisions about allocation of keyworkers should be based on how best to meet the needs of individual residents.
- Ensure new staff have time to become familiar with residents and their care plans and needs.
- Ensure good communication between all the professionals and organisations involved.
- Do not rely on families to explain the change to residents.
- Put effort into explaining the changes to residents with dementia (for example using photographs and small group discussions over coffee). It may be useful to create a storybook with photographs and so on that staff and families can use with residents to reiterate what will be happening.
- Set up residents' rooms as far as possible to mirror what they left behind.
- Ensure new arrangements support the maintenance of existing friendships between residents as far as possible.
- Ensure that a familiar person is accompanying each resident on every step of the way.

Box 1.5: Opening a new dementia care home

- Build in plenty of time for preparation, at least 18 months.
- Develop operational policies while the home is being built.
- Negotiate early with community services about the levels of support that will be needed from their staff.
- Have the staff team appointed several weeks before opening to allow for induction (see Chapter 4).
- Ensure staff recruitment is phased to match the schedule for admitting residents and 'opening' units within the home.
- Ensure the recruitment of some experienced staff, who can immediately work effectively and help with induction and training; balance experienced staff with staff who are new to care work and who can more easily be moulded into the ways of the new home.
- Ensure there is budget provision for an induction period.
- Adapt standard induction programmes (see Chapter 4) to ensure that, before residents arrive, the staff group has enough time to get to know the building and its equipment and to rehearse basic working practices.
- Build in plenty of time for team building and staff support.
- Do not overextend the induction period prior to opening: staff can become bored and demotivated when they are not able to 'get on with the real job'.
- Appoint maintenance and administrative staff before opening.
- Stagger admissions; assume at least a month and possibly up to nine months before operating at full capacity.
- Consider carefully how the first admissions will be handled; remember that, because this is a new venture, staff and relatives may have more than the usual anxieties.
- Consider how some 'public relations' activities with the local community might lay good foundations for future involvement.

Box 1.6: Setting up a new dementia care home involving relocation

- Think carefully about when to involve staff, relatives and residents; it is important to involve people from an early stage but if issues are raised too early there may be too many uncertainties for it to be constructive.
- Involve people from the reprovided home in every detail from the stage of selecting the site onwards.
- Keep relatives informed and involved (for example, through open days, formal meetings, individual discussions and newsletters).
- Be aware of families' anxieties and that they will experience the timescale very differently from managers; for example, progress will seem slow to many and it is important to keep communication going even through the 'nothing much happening' phases of building work.
- Keep staff informed and involved throughout.
- Make sure that staffing issues are dealt with in a timely, fair and sensitive manner. This will involve issues of terms and conditions of service, changes in job descriptions, training and development needs and people's emotional reactions to the change.
- Spend time with staff individually to discuss the change, job opportunities, their individual concerns and so on.
- Begin to develop staff teams well before the move, for example, through small group workshops.
- Match keyworkers with residents. Maintain existing relationships where possible and allow time for new relationships to become established well before the move.
- As far as possible have residents and staff together in the same groups before, during and after the move.
- Assume it may take a couple of months for residents to settle.
- Allow for additional staff over the period of the move (one study home had triple staffing for one week, double for 6-8 weeks, tapering to normal after about 12 weeks).

The move
- Arrange transport to suit individual residents (after discussion with keyworkers and families).
- Have an 'open house' for families over the period of the move (for example, set aside a lounge for them to use).
- Have the new building cleaned and all furniture in place before residents arrive.
- Phase the move over several days or even weeks.

2 Management matters

Introduction

Supportive management and good leadership are crucial for good quality dementia care[39]. This chapter examines:

- values and principles in practice
- management structures
- the tasks, characteristics and recruitment of good dementia care home managers
- quality management
- staff management
- involving residents and relatives in management
- managing links with external services.

It concludes by commenting on the importance of management development.

Values and principles in practice

Good dementia care requires managers to ensure that the values and principles which we identified in Chapter 1 are translated into everyday practice. This does not necessarily mean that staff are able to quote mission and value statements – it does mean that the core values are reflected in the way staff describe their work and go about their daily activities. Box 2.1 lists the factors that managers variously identified as central to ensuring that organisational culture and day-to-day practice are permeated by the values and principles of good dementia care.

Management structures

The role of parent organisations

Some homes are independently owned but many are part of larger organisations and the management of the individual home is then shaped by the parent provider organisation's management style. Parent organisations vary in the extent to which they allow individual homes to have autonomy[40]. In our case studies there was considerable consensus that parent organisations should give home managers a good deal of autonomy. This accords with evidence that levels of satisfaction in managers is linked to their feeling of having a high level of autonomy. In new homes especially, managers need to feel that they can try out new ideas and that they will be supported in doing this.

Box 2.1: Translating values and principles into practice

- Be clear about the home's core values and principles.
- Be clear about goals that are in accord with these values and principles.
- Ensure staff induction emphasises the values and principles.
- Ensure core values and principles are reinforced through staff training and development.
- Ensure management and systems support staff in day-to-day implementation of the values and principles.
- Provide good leadership that demonstrates the values and principles.

The larger case study organisations all provided new homes with operational policy manuals with which they were expected to comply. Managers in smaller organisations generally had a much greater role in developing operational policies. Reporting arrangements for home managers varied with the size of the parent organisation, particularly in the level of formality and use of standardised and numerical returns. In larger organisations, the home manager generally reported regularly to a line manager who had professional and general management responsibility. The line manager's professional expertise was important in picking up any care practice problems in the home. In small organisations, the senior managers were usually general managers and the home manager therefore carried the main responsibility for professional care.

One of the benefits of having dementia care homes in large provider organisations is that it is then feasible to have specialist dementia advice at senior management level. Two of our study organisations had a dementia care specialist manager based in headquarters. In one organisation the dementia care specialist was the line manager for the home manager. In the other organisation, a regional manager undertook the line management role with the dementia care specialist providing the home with advice and support. The specialist dementia managers in both organisations advised on staff recruitment, induction and training; provided information about best practice in dementia care; and facilitated networking between dementia services.

One of the issues for home managers is the extent to which they feel that they and their organisation share the same values and priorities. The tensions that were most often mentioned in our study were in relation to the relative importance attached to quality of care and financial performance. On the whole, home managers accepted the economic realities of running the organisation as long as they could remain confident that there would be no unreasonable stinting on the resources needed for resident care. A number of managers compared their present organisation favourably with their experience elsewhere of residents being deprived of expensive essentials or inexpensive, but nonetheless important, comforts.

Box 2.2 summarises some of the ways in which provider organisations can be good 'parents' to specialist dementia care homes.

Internal care home management

The management arrangements for each of the case study homes are shown in Table 2.1.

Box 2.2: Dementia care homes: some features of good parent provider organisations

- Ensure there is a strong commitment to excellence in dementia care at all levels of the organisation.
- Ensure that everyone, from care staff to the chief executive, shares the same understanding of the organisation's values and purposes.
- Ensure clarity of roles and responsibilities between the organisation's centre and the individual home.
- Give home managers as much autonomy as possible in managing their units.
- Ensure home managers feel supported in their work.
- Ensure home managers have the resources to do the job.
- Convey to managers and their staff that the organisation values them and listens to their views.
- Ensure a strong commitment to staff development at all levels in the organisation.
- Give staff a sense of ownership and sharing in the organisation's success.
- Recognise the contribution that other services make to the success of the home.
- Demonstrate a commitment to being 'trail blazing'.
- Demonstrate a commitment to continuous learning and development.

Table 2.1: Management arrangements in the case study homes

Home	Structure	Management
A	36 beds in 4 units	Manager, assistant and 4 shift team leaders (who cover the whole home and are all RMNs)
B	36 beds in 3 units	Manager, deputy and 2 assistants
C	60 beds in 4 units	Manager, deputy, part-time care team manager for each unit plus 2 full-time care managers (one for each floor); night care manager is additional
D	24 beds in 3 units	Manager and deputy; deputy has clinical lead and works some shifts as part of the care rota; 2 trained nurses work across the 3 units
E	72 beds in 3 units	Manager plus 3 care managers (responsible for all systems in a unit as well as management across the home); senior care staff on each unit
F	23 beds in 3 units	Manager, deputy
G	60 beds in 2 units	Manager, deputy and 1 nursing sister or staff nurse in each unit

Care home managers

This section focuses on the role of the home manager. This is not intended to imply that other grades of manager are less important. Deputies, assistants, shift team leaders, unit managers and so on all have vital roles. The skills and attributes needed for these posts vary depending, among other things, on the specific post, the size of the home and the expectations of the home manager. Compared with the home manager, these managers are more involved in the detail of the day-to-day work of the home. Their influence in maintaining the culture of the home and high standards of care practice should not be underestimated. Many of the points that we make below about the skills and attributes required of home managers, and about management development, apply equally to other members of the management team. Indeed, it is the functioning of the management team that is crucial in determining quality of care[41].

Key tasks

The role of care home manager combines professional care management and business management. Within the sector, there is consensus that to guarantee quality the manager's role in care provision should have priority over their business role[42]. Managers themselves generally see 'organising staff' as their principal role and think others should deal with financial issues[42]. In our study homes, the home managers were required to pay attention to business concerns but overall responsibility for the health of the business lay with the parent organisation[42]. The home managers were therefore able to focus their main attention on issues related to staffing and care provision.

The nature of the manager's task varies depending on the size of the home and also on whether the manager is an owner manager or a manager within a corporate organisation[42]. Our case studies show how the management task also varies depending on the nature and size of the corporate organisation. For example, the managers of Homes D and F, whose parent organisations had more limited experience of care home provision, had a greater than usual role in establishing new management systems. In addition, in small, as compared with large organisations, the home manager's role may be rather isolated as there is limited scope for internal networking.

Recruitment and selection of home managers

Processes

Managers in our study homes were appointed in various ways:

- two were already working for the parent organisation
- two were effectively 'head hunted' as they already had a good reputation in services in the area
- three were appointed through open competition.

Depending on the local employment market, advertisements for management posts generally need to be placed regionally if not nationally.

Qualifications and experience

The qualifications and experience of care home managers vary considerably. Within the sector there is consensus that managers of care homes for older people should have[42]:

- client-specific skills (and if transferring from working with another client group they should have further training)
- management and supervisory experience in care homes (approximately 2½-3 years' minimum experience in managing a care home and in working with older people)
- a 'working with older persons' qualification
- a management-relevant qualification.

For homes that require the manager to be a qualified nurse, it is important that the qualification is appropriate to the post (for example, an RMN for a dementia care home) and accompanied by extensive relevant experience[43].

There is ongoing debate about the respective value of nursing and social care qualifications for care home management. The sector generally values nursing qualifications more than social care qualifications but it also thinks there should be good social work skills in homes[44]. It has been suggested that the ideal solution to such professional boundary issues would be a new form of generic worker who would combine the skills of a range of social and health professions[45]. This could certainly fit well with the requirements of high quality dementia care. In the absence of such generically qualified workers, two of the study homes went some way to addressing the problem by having a manager who was dual qualified in social care and in nursing. Other managers' qualifications included: RMN (1); RGN (1); RMN and RGN (1); social care (2).

For dementia care homes, managers should have experience of managing care for people with dementia and should have up-to-date understanding of dementia[46]. Our case studies suggest that it is also important that managers have had frontline experience of dementia care provision. Several managers said this type of experience gave them credibility in the eyes of staff. Moreover, they felt confident and comfortable that they were not asking staff to do anything they had not done themselves.

Skills and attributes

Whatever the qualifications and professional background of managers, they need a range of skills[47] in such areas as:

- individual and group care practice
- working within the regulatory and legal framework
- business strategy
- finance and property management
- policy implementation
- staff management
- organisational change management
- self-management.

The level of skills required will vary depending on the type of home and the tasks required within the organisation's management arrangements (see page 16). Moreover, the skills and personal attributes needed for managing a new home are different from those required for managing a well-established home. Senior managers in the provider organisations in our study identified important criteria to use when appointing a manager to set up a new dementia care home (see Box 2.3).

Box 2.3: Criteria for appointing managers for new dementia care homes

Managers should ideally have:
- a strong interest in dementia care
- a track record in dementia care development
- the ability to set up new systems
- the ability to develop good relationships with a range of people
- expertise in teambuilding
- resilience in coping with problems, frustrations and setbacks
- commitment to promoting the unique aspects of care for people with dementia
- the ambition to be 'trail blazing'
- a flair for innovation
- commitment to setting and maintaining high standards from day one – 'to start as they mean to go on'
- personal qualities of leadership
- prior experience of setting up a home or similar service.

> **Box 2.4: Characteristics of good dementia care home managers**
>
> Managers should:
> - be available to staff
> - have good communication skills and have an easy, comfortable style of interaction
> - have a non-hierarchical approach, for example one manager explained, "I don't like to be called the boss"
> - be clear about standards and expectations
> - have a 'light touch' but the capacity to be firm when necessary to achieve good standards
> - deal with difficult issues 'quietly' within a 'no blame' culture
> - be committed to teamwork and to including all staff in the home as members of the team
> - be committed to knowing, valuing and trusting staff
> - be open, honest and fair with staff
> - be prepared to go 'on the floor' and provide a role model
> - lead using reason and explanation rather than position power
> - be committed to self-development and to passing on their expertise to others, including 'bringing on' other staff in a management capacity
> - be creative, innovative and forward looking
> - balance idealism and realism
> - recognise their own and their staff's limitations
> - have a strong focus on knowing their residents and working in their interests, for example one manager explained, "... I refer back to what is right for the resident. If I do that I always get what I want".

Management and leadership style

We know at least some of the components of good leadership and management in dementia care settings. These include:

- fostering a 'creative culture'[48]
- leading by example[49]
- setting clear goals[50]
- planning and advocating for the unit[50]
- encouraging and stimulating innovation (and accepting that there are risks that go with this)[50]
- a non-hierarchical management approach[51].

The personal styles of the managers in our case study homes varied: some managers had a strong, extrovert and 'charismatic' style while others had a quieter but nonetheless effective style. This accords with research that suggests that while charismatic leadership is desirable it is by no means essential[52].

Despite some differences in personal style, there was much in common between the managers in the characteristics that they and their staff identified as being important. These characteristics are summarised in Box 2.4. There are many similarities between this list and other sources of advice about good care home management[53].

Quality management

Quality requirements and systems

Specialist dementia care homes are required to meet minimum standards for care homes[54]. However, achieving good practice involves more than that. Quality systems are widely advocated as a valuable approach to improving quality, although only a very small proportion of care homes use formal systems[55]. A variety of quality management systems are available for use in care homes for older people. Different systems focus on different aspects of provision and the value of a package must be assessed in relation to the purpose for which it is to be used[56].

Although the need for quality assurance in dementia care has been long recognised[57], there is no one widely used system specifically designed for this purpose. Dementia care mapping (DCM)[58], which uses detailed observations to assess residents' well-being, has been found to be useful in dealing with some aspects of quality management (see below). The Alzheimer's Society's work on producing care standards uses a rather different approach[59]. More detailed discussions of quality issues and systems in residential care generally[60], and dementia care[61] more specifically, are available.

Quality management in practice

The homes in our study had a variety of quality management arrangements. Four homes had no formal internal quality systems but used a range of techniques to ensure high standards. In Homes C and G there were regular visits from a senior headquarters-based manager who 'went round' the home. This was supplemented by routine reports to headquarters quantifying aspects of practice and resource use. Managers used their own informal monitoring, for example one home manager described regular 'spot checking'. In two smaller homes (D and F), the managers were happy that they had a sound approach to ensuring good quality care. The factors that they identified as being central to their approach were very similar to the factors that were important in the homes that operated the more formal quality systems described below. One of these homes had decided to develop a more formal audit process to demonstrate quality to purchasers and to provide 'cover' from a legal standpoint.

One of the homes with a more formal system – Home E – participated in a local authority scheme that gave a top-up payment per resident for homes meeting certain standards based on an annual inspection and the production of specified evidence. The parent organisation's own quality system involved the home undertaking quality surveys on topics identified by the manager as being important. Another home – Home A – was part of its parent organisation's extensive quality system founded on a Japanese approach called Toazen. Key elements of this included:

- corporate goals set by the parent organisation in different areas of service operation, for example, quality, cost, service delivery and 'delights' for residents (see Chapter 3)
- monthly paper returns to headquarters quantifying a range of aspects of practice and resource use
- 'KAIZEN' which involves identifying problems, identifying what should ideally be happening, and bringing all managers and staff involved together to generate ideas and 'bite-size' actions to make this happen
- 'Quality Quest' which involves the home in benchmarking itself against other services inside and outside the organisation
- a 'Buzz Words' suggestion scheme that encourages staff, relatives and residents to put forward ideas for improvements.

Home B was also part of its parent organisation's comprehensive quality management system. This system placed a strong emphasis on staff empowerment and valuing staff. The overall approach was to avoid a paper chase and to treat the quality system as a tool and not an end in itself. The system included: a quality manual setting out policies, procedures and standards across a wide range of aspects of care home operation; and, internal staff audit teams assessing performance in specified areas and feeding back the results to the home manager and ultimately to the parent organisation.

Quality management issues

There are some issues about how dementia care homes fit into corporate quality and performance management systems whose standards and audit processes are not designed to fit dementia care. A key issue is how audit teams should include the views of residents (a standard aspect of much good quality auditing) when they have dementia. One home was exploring the use of observational techniques to obtain the residents' perspective rather than the direct questions that would be asked of residents in the organisation's other care environments. Another issue is the use of quality measures designed for care environments with residents who are more able. Staff and managers of one home felt that if they focused on achieving some of the performance targets set by their organisation they would inappropriately distort the care of their residents.

There is also the issue of what constitutes appropriate measures of quality in dementia care. One manager described how the staff group had had much discussion about how to measure success in caring for people with dementia who may respond with indifference or aggression to even the best care efforts. Three of the organisations had experience of DCM[62] through working on projects which involved external people using DCM to assess the home's care practice. Two managers had been trained in DCM and had used this to assess quality. They explained that they liked the principles on which DCM is founded but felt it had some limitations insofar as it identified problems but not necessarily how to solve them. Their general view was that DCM could be useful but that, in the words of one manager, "it's just a tool and only as good as the person using it".

It was clear from our discussions with managers and staff that if quality systems are to be effective in influencing practice they must make sense to staff, and staff must have ownership of the processes and outcomes. Managers need to judge carefully how far to push staff to meet performance targets. In one home, for example, it was clear that, while some staff were committed to the quality system, a good number were sceptical of its value.

Most importantly the case studies show that while a formal, structured and comprehensive quality management system has benefits, it is not essential to good quality care. What is essential is management commitment to pursuit of quality and management recognition that quality is dependent on good staff.

Box 2.5 summarises the important lessons identified in this section.

Box 2.5: How to achieve quality

- Have a clear philosophy and ensure that all staff understand the philosophy and work to it.
- Ensure good management–staff communication and relationships based on managers being approachable and not threatening to staff.
- Work on the basis that there is always scope for improvement.
- Be willing to respond to criticisms and suggestions. As one manager put it: "I put my hand up if something is not right, and try to address it".
- Ensure that management has strong expectations and standards, and communicates these to staff.
- Ensure that managers spend time 'on the floor'.
- Promote staff education and training, including dementia-specific inputs.
- Adapt any general quality and performance targets to take account of the specifics of dementia care.
- Ensure that the perspectives of residents with dementia are incorporated into quality management.
- Ensure that managers and staff have ownership of quality systems.
- Ensure that the quality system values all staff by allowing everyone to raise quality issues.
- Treat quality systems as a means to an end (that is, good quality care) and not an end in themselves.
- Use quality systems that involve realistic time commitments and avoid volumes of paperwork.

Staff management

Chapter 4 deals in more detail with staffing issues. Here we focus on the managers' perspective on three aspects of staff management: communication in the organisation, managing the staff as a group and supervision as a means of performance management.

Communication in the organisation

Several parent organisations and individual homes stressed the importance of staff having a sense of ownership, feeling involved in the organisation and knowing that their views mattered. Achieving this requires good communication with staff. The communication strategies used in study homes varied according to the size and structure of the homes and their parent organisations. They included:

- organisation-wide and home-based newsletters for staff and residents
- unit staff meetings within homes
- shift team staff meetings within homes
- monthly cascade of information from manager to units through 'team briefing' of a representative from each unit
- meetings of the home's management team
- meetings with managers across a number of homes in the organisation.

In one home there were few staff meetings because the manager's style was to work individually rather than with groups. This worked well because it was a small home, because the manager was a very good communicator and because he invested considerable time and energy in ensuring good communication.

Managing the staff group

Several managers talked about the importance of handling the personal dynamics and emotional aspects of the staff group. One manager talked about there being two approaches to running a home. In the first approach, staff do their job and have little emotional contact with colleagues. In the second approach, staff care about each other and support each other. The manager argued that this second approach, when combined with an open, non-blaming management style, has the advantage that the manager can feel confident about high standards of care as staff effectively 'police' each other.

Managers must pay attention to the relationships between different staff groups, especially between qualified and unqualified staff. In our study homes, unqualified staff usually appreciated the advice and support available from qualified colleagues. However, they also felt that their role and contribution was sometimes constrained and not fully valued by qualified staff, especially nursing staff[63]. Since good person-centred dementia care is dependent on all staff feeling supported and valued as members of the care team, managers need to ensure that any potential role confusion and frustration are avoided[64] by having appropriate, and not necessarily traditional, role definitions accepted in the staff group.

Staff performance and support

> The system of supervision is the heart of a training and development strategy, and the key to the maintenance of high standards in the long-term. (Kitwood and Woods, 1996[65], p 16)

All of our study homes used supervision as a means of performance management and staff support. The way homes organised supervision varied, in part influenced by the size of the home. Supervision arrangements included:

- all staff having monthly supervision sessions with either the manager or deputy manager
- the manager supervising the qualified staff (and the chef, gardener and handyperson) with the qualified staff in turn each supervising several care staff
- a cascade of supervision from area manager through home manager, unit managers, senior care staff, to care staff and support service staff, including housekeepers, chefs and so on.

Several managers described the supportive aspects of supervision and stressed that supervision sessions were confidential and often very emotional.

In a couple of our case study homes, internal support for staff was supplemented by arrangements for individual, external confidential counselling for staff at their own request. In another home, the manager mentioned that the chaplain willingly and ably provided confidential staff support. In general, these additional support mechanisms were not much used and staff did not see this as an essential arrangement as long as management encouraged staff to come forward with any difficulties or concerns. As staff in one home put it: "It is drummed into us – come and see us [managers] if you have a problem".

Home managers in our study talked very little about staff disciplinary policies and procedures. Their approach to maintaining high standards of conduct was instead characterised by:

- ensuring staff internalised the high standards of the home
- using peer pressure to ensure conformity to high standards
- having an approachable style that encouraged staff to come forward if they had problems
- using their own 'personal antennae' to pick up on any problems
- having a high level of staff respect for their authority.

Home A, which was generally the most 'systems oriented' of our case studies, was the only one in which we gained a sense of staff disciplinary rules operating explicitly in day-to-day practice. For example, in this home a strong emphasis on staff spending time with residents was accompanied by explicit, and quite strictly applied rules about staff break times and time-keeping in general. The manager in this home explained that its approach followed the Samurai disciplinary code (in line with the organisation's Japanese quality management system): "respect the strong, support the weak and cut off the heads of the wicked".

Involving residents and relatives in management

The involvement of residents and relatives in individual care matters is discussed in Chapter 3. Here we deal with how residents and relatives are enabled to influence the management and general life of the home. Meaningful consultation with care home residents is often difficult to achieve[66] and homes should use a variety of means to ensure that residents' views are taken into account[67]. The challenge is even greater when residents have dementia.

Three study homes had regular residents' meetings for the purposes of consultation; in two homes, relatives also attended the meetings. The three homes that held residents' meetings all had units for physically frail residents; residents with dementia were only involved in the meetings in one of these homes. The home that had consultation with residents with dementia held a regular meeting, conducted by the manager, in the dementia unit. Not all residents with dementia were able to participate, and the level of comment elicited was quite limited. However, including the dementia unit in the home's round of consultative meetings was seen to be symbolically important in confirming the value and rights of residents with dementia.

Limited consultation with residents with dementia reflects prevailing practice in care homes. However, we now know that people with dementia, even people with advanced dementia and significant communication difficulties, have views about services that they are able to express[68]. We also know that care staff can enable people with dementia to express their views if they are given the time, opportunity and support to develop individualised approaches to communication. We should therefore expect that specialist dementia care homes will rise to the challenge of making consultation with residents an integral feature of their services.

All of the study homes held meetings with relatives to keep them up to date with any developments in the home, to provide them with an opportunity to discuss any general concerns and to allow them to make suggestions about the home and its services. These meetings took a variety of forms and varied very considerably in how regularly they were held. One home, for example, had an annual meeting attended by the home manager, senior staff and senior managers from the parent organisation. Another home held a six-weekly 'relatives' forum' which the manager of the home attended. The differences in the form and frequency of the meetings were related to their functions; some consultation meetings were also used as social events and to provide informal support for relatives. Whichever approach is taken, managers need to make efforts to overcome the tendency for relatives simply to express satisfaction with the service rather than come forward with more detailed and constructive criticisms.

For consultation meetings to be successful, it is important that:

- relatives are given plenty of notice of the meeting
- meetings are held at times that are likely to be convenient to relatives
- meetings are conducted with enough informality to encourage relatives to participate and enough formality to convey that what they say will be taken seriously
- managers make it clear that they are open to criticism and that they expect relatives to identify areas for improvement
- managers demonstrate that they are committed to acting in response to criticisms and suggestions.

Managing links with external services

Quality care depends not only on good management of the home but also on having multidisciplinary links with a wide range of other health services[69] as well as social care services and other facilities. The main services and facilities that are needed are listed in Tables 2.2a and 2.2b, alongside comments from our study homes about the management issues involved.

Homes need to consider carefully when it is better to have services come into the home and when it is better to have residents going out to use ordinary services. Relatives' views on this matter do not always accord with staff views. For example, one home encouraged residents to visit their GP with a relative. But the relatives did not like it when, as they put it, the resident, "is just another patient in the waiting room". Relatives

Table 2.2a: Use of external health services

Service	Comment
General medicine	Homes reported that GPs vary in their knowledge and interest in dementia care. Most homes felt it important to have a 'friendly' or 'preferred' practice with which they had developed particularly good links. All homes enabled residents to have the local GP of their choice. A few homes had a 'contract' with a local GP practice to visit the home regularly to provide general advice and occasional staff training.
Psychiatry and neurology	Contact was generally limited to a few residents who remained under the ongoing care of a consultant, usually in old age psychiatry (or neurology for some younger residents with dementia). Only one home reported regular visits by a consultant; but none of the homes had any problems in linking with these services.
Community nursing (for example psychiatric, continence, palliative care and district nurses)	This was generally arranged through the resident's GP and provided by local NHS trusts. It is a very important service for homes, particularly those without qualified nursing staff. Links are generally excellent.
Acute hospitalisation	Acute problems were generally well treated but people with dementia often experienced detrimental side effects from poor general care, for example, inappropriate psychotropic medication; unnecessary catheterisation; immobility and pressure sores; inadequate fluid and food intake. More than one home sent staff into acute wards with residents to help people with eating, washing and so on.
Chiropody	This was sometimes provided by the NHS, sometimes by a private agency and sometimes both visited homes regularly.
Dentistry	Generally local dental practices visited homes on request. Annual checks are desirable as well as treatment as required.
Optometry	Generally a local 'high street' optician visited homes on request.
Audiology	Access to audiology and hearing aid clinics is important, although it was seldom mentioned in our case studies.
Occupational therapy	Occupational therapy was not extensively used. NHS access is variable in different localities and homes sometimes addressed inadequacies in NHS services by employing their own therapists.
Physiotherapy	Physiotherapy was not extensively used. NHS access was variable in different localities and homes sometimes addressed inadequacies in NHS services by employing their own therapists.
Dietetics	A dietician was only used by one home in which the organisation was working closely with the dietician in the local NHS trust to develop a menu plan that would ensure good levels of nutrition for people with dementia.
Speech and language therapy	Speech and language therapy was not used by our case study homes, but may be needed for some people with dementia.
Complementary therapies	Aromatherapy was provided by trained staff in two homes and reflexology in one home.

Table 2.2b: Use of external social care services and community facilities

Service	Comments
Social services	Social services contact was generally around the time of admission with little routine involvement after the review of placement six weeks after admission. Homes often need to supplement the care manager's assessment with their own assessment and information gathering.
Religious	Some homes had a chaplain. Most had contact with a range of local churches to provide pastoral visits and conduct services in the home. It is important to ensure that residents of all faiths have access to religious contacts and services.
Library	In some areas local libraries delivered books, including large print and 'talking books'. In one area the local library provided 'reminiscence boxes' about every three weeks filled with materials related to a particular period.
Hairdressing	Usually a hairdresser visited regularly to provide services on an individual private basis. Hairdressing sessions were a popular social focus in a number of homes.
Shopping	A couple of homes provided a trolley service once or twice a week from which residents could buy small items such as toiletries and confectionery. Most shopping for residents was done by relatives and, occasionally, staff. Some homes made considerable efforts to take residents with dementia out for shopping.
Telephone	A telephone point in each resident's room is desirable to allow use of a private telephone. For residents without their own telephone there should be a cordless telephone readily available.

thought that the GP should be asked to visit the home. Some relatives went so far as to suggest that it would be better to have a GP for the home rather than residents having their own choice of GP. This view was counter to the general desire of homes to avoid 'block treatment' by visiting professionals. One manager specifically expressed concern about the quality of the service provided by some commercial companies (such as some opticians) coming in to treat 'captive' customer groups.

Management development

Management development has received little attention in the care home sector[70]. The organisations in this study all recognised that good management is essential for good care. Their management development commitment generally took two forms: line management support and financial support for managers to do degree courses or other advanced training programmes. One organisation provided management foundation courses for senior nursing staff but did not yet have programmes for home managers. Another organisation had recognised the need for a more coherent and comprehensive approach and was in the process of reviewing its management development strategy. Overall, management development was somewhat piecemeal. Providers of dementia care homes should address management development as a priority.

3

Care matters

Introduction

It is not the purpose of this chapter to provide detailed practice guidance; that is available elsewhere[71]. This chapter simply aims to brief managers who are new to the dementia field or who want an update on current thinking about key issues in dementia care.

Person-centred care

Chapter 1 describes the essential values and principles of good dementia care homes. Many of these are encapsulated within the notion of person-centred care. All of the homes in our study were committed to person-centred care and some homes explicitly linked their approach with ideas about 'the new culture of dementia care'[72].

Central to person-centred dementia care is the concept of 'personhood'[72]. Maintaining the individual with dementia's personhood involves fostering their sense of identity and worth. Thus, in interacting with people with dementia we must[73]:

- be honest, encouraging, accepting, empowering and inclusive
- treat them as adults
- avoid pejorative labels
- let them set the pace
- validate their feelings and experiences
- recognise their unique humanity
- treat them as people not as objects.

Knowing the individual

Good dementia care must be tailored to the biography and interests, likes and dislikes, values and personality of each person. It can be difficult for staff to know what is important for individual residents with dementia: for example, how they would like their lives to be arranged and their care to be provided. In the day-to-day bustle of 'getting on with the job', there is always a tendency for staff to resort to what they think a resident wants. It is important therefore that staff ideas are founded on as much knowledge of the resident as possible. Also, staff ideas about what residents want must be reviewed regularly; otherwise residents risk being 'typecast' even in small things such as 'she always has porridge'.

Life story books have become well accepted as a useful means of getting to know people with dementia and of keeping a record of the myriad things that make them a unique person[74]. Our study homes applied and adapted the life story book idea in several ways. One home compiled a 'book of life' for each resident which was put together by the keyworker with assistance from relatives and the person with dementia. The 'book of life' included photographs, personal documents, mementoes and a diary of daily social activities. For staff, the book was a powerful tool, reminding them about the resident's individuality and reinforcing relatives' views about how care should be provided. Another home used 'storyboards' that were produced in a similar way but then mounted on the wall in the resident's room. This ensured that the information was always readily available to prompt conversation on topics of interest to the resident and to remind staff of the resident's preferences. A third home developed 'lifestyle profiles' for each resident. The profiles used knowledge of the person's personal history, behaviour, likes and dislikes to describe their preferred daily and weekly 'lifestyle' in the home. This approach recognises that, like most people, people with dementia need some routine and structure to their days[75] and that, in care homes, such routines should be based on each individual's preferred lifestyle rather than the needs of the organisation.

Some advice about how to achieve person-centred practice, based on examples that we encountered during our study visits, is listed in Box 3.1. Achieving person-centred care requires a strong management commitment. Staff need to be empowered to move beyond the tasks and routines of care provision to develop care that is imaginative and sensitive to individual residents.

Communicating with people with dementia

Good communication with people with dementia is essential for person-centred dementia care[76]. If staff have time, patience and commitment they can achieve much better levels of communication than has generally been assumed possible.

However, this is also one of the biggest challenges for specialist dementia care homes. Communication and interaction needs to be addressed as it occurs throughout everyday life and activity in the home. It is important that all staff, including domestic and catering staff, are involved in the home's efforts to achieve good communication. Guidance on the skills and techniques of good communication is available[77]. Managers must be committed to ensuring that staff have the training and support needed to develop their skills and practice in communicating with people with dementia. But good communication requires more than this – managers must be committed to promoting a culture in which communication and interaction is valued as core care work.

Box 3.1: Person-centred care: how to achieve good practice

- Encourage residents and relatives to personalise the resident's room, particularly to reflect something of the style of the person with dementia's earlier home.
- Involve residents and relatives in choosing the colour scheme for the room.
- Tailor care to individual preferences and familiar routines, for example, natural waking times, preferences about rising, preferences about baths or showers and when to have them.
- Consider having 'delight goals' (an idea from Home A) that involve arranging for the person with dementia to do some of the special things that they 'always wanted to do'.
- Provide for individual musical tastes (for example, by arranging for residents to spend time in their room listening to their preferred music).
- Provide for individual tastes in food and preferences about mealtimes (see page 31).
- Pay attention to detail in residents' dress, for example that skirt length is appropriate.
- Provide 'pampering' in personal care, for example, using bath essence, spa baths, hair brushing, hand massage.
- Match keyworker and other staff to residents' preferences (for example, male or female, quiet or extrovert personality).
- Provide good physical healthcare.
- Get to know and respond to each individual's whims.
- Accommodate important features of the resident's previous life (examples included someone having a greenhouse set up in the garden and finding space for someone's beloved baby grand piano even when the resident could no longer play).
- Provide occupation and stimulation that is relevant to the individual's past and current interests.
- Work at the resident's own pace and do not rush them.
- Learn little details about residents that can help in tailoring care.
- Spend time one-to-one with residents.
- Encourage residents to express preferences and make choices whenever possible.
- Use appropriate touch and expressions of affection.
- Respect the privacy of the individual's room.

Behaviour that presents a challenge for staff

At times, people with dementia in care homes may behave in ways that staff find difficult and stressful, for example by being aggressive or agitated or resisting 'care'. It used to be assumed that such behaviour was simply 'a result of the dementia' and it was managed accordingly, often through the use of medication. More recently our thinking has become more sophisticated. First, we now know that it is important to understand the behaviour as part of the person with dementia's attempts to deal with the world that they are experiencing and to communicate something about that experience to others. Thus, the behaviour that staff experience as difficult may be an expression of the person with dementia's feelings of, for example, anger or frustration. Second, we know that staff vary in the extent to which they perceive behaviour as 'challenging' and in how they respond to it[78]. Third, we know that staff use a variety of strategies to cope with such behaviour and that these are often unconstructive in that they stifle residents' communication and expression, and lead to further 'problems'[79]. Guidance is available on best practice in responding to 'challenging behaviour'[80].

Managers in our study homes generally claimed to have lower than usual levels of 'difficult to manage' behaviour in their homes as well as low use of medication for the control of behaviour. They attributed this to the provision of good person-centred care in general and more specifically to their efforts to minimise residents' distress by:

- creating a calm and relaxed environment
- giving people space to walk about so that they do not feel confined and restricted
- ensuring that people are neither bored nor over-stimulated
- pre-empting problems by developing staff communication skills to enable them to understand what the person with dementia is feeling and trying to express
- pre-empting problems by 'knowing the person' and knowing how to respond in situations that are potentially distressing for them.

Despite these strategies, staff in all of the homes experienced some behaviour that they regarded as difficult. In all cases, their approach in such circumstances was a problem solving one. They tried to understand the behaviour from the perspective of the person with dementia and to respond by adapting the environment or care practice to better meet the individual's needs.

Managers of dementia homes should ensure that staff training includes good practice in managing so-called 'challenging behaviour'[81]. However, such training is of most value when it is part of a broad management strategy for good person-centred care[82].

Spirituality and sexuality

Spirituality and sexuality are core dimensions of personal identity and must be addressed in person-centred care[83]. Staff and managers often find work in these areas difficult because of the strong social values, expectations and inhibitions that surround them.

Sexuality was not raised as a major issue in our case study homes but issues are likely to arise in dementia care (for example, residents may develop sexual relationships; some people with dementia become disinhibited). Managers must be prepared to respond sensitively and appropriately[84].

Spirituality was particularly significant in a couple of our study homes whose parent provider organisation had an explicitly religious foundation. Other homes made provision to enable residents to maintain religious observances but generally attention to spirituality was much less evident. A variety of approaches are suggested for meeting spiritual needs in care homes generally[85] and in dementia care more specifically[86].

Care planning

Admissions

The care process begins with a referral for admission. The assessment practices of social services care managers prior to admission vary in nature and quality, so assessment by the home is very important. The process of admission to a care home needs always to be handled carefully but even more so for people with dementia. Drawing on the literature[87] and our case studies, we identify important aspects of good admissions practice in Box 3.2:

> ### Box 3.2: Good admissions practice
>
> - Ensure that senior staff from the home have assessed the resident against the home's own clear admission criteria (see also Chapter 1).
> - If possible, base the assessment on a visit to the potential resident's own home.
> - Ensure that the person with dementia is involved in the process and that they understand and consent to the decision as fully as possible.
> - Assure relatives and friends of the importance of their continued involvement in the resident's life.
> - Begin the process of 'getting to know the person' by finding out as much as possible from carers, relatives, friends, other services and the resident themselves.
> - Do as much as possible to ease the transition for the resident by bringing along familiar objects and involving familiar people.
> - Respond to the emotional needs of the relatives, for example, feelings of loss or guilt.
> - Recognise that a resident with dementia will take extra time to get to know their new environment.

Care plans

Most care homes have care planning arrangements, but there are often significant gaps between the rhetoric and reality of care planning[88]. Care plans (in the form of paper records) are only one element of a broader care planning process. If we are to ensure good care we need to focus on the processes and outcomes of care planning and not just on the structures and documentation.

Care planning for people with dementia needs to be based on 'knowing the person' (see page 25). A range of approaches to individualising care plans can include:

- life story work
- 24-hour diaries
- activity diaries
- interviews with family members
- small group staff discussions about individual residents.

Staff often find life story work rewarding. Approaches that are highly paper-based can be daunting for some staff[89].

Care planning needs to focus on the retained abilities of the person with dementia otherwise there is a tendency towards unwarranted assumptions of disability and the promotion of dependency. Care plans should also be comprehensive in addressing the full range of each individual's physical and mental health needs.

Care plans necessarily focus on the individual resident but in doing so they should not neglect the social relationships that exist in any group of residents since, "Good quality of care must include promoting good relationships and opportunities to interact positively"[90]. This is a particularly important consideration in homes that have small units because in these settings residents have less opportunity to choose their companions.

Only a few care planning systems have been developed specifically for dementia care, some in NHS continuing care settings[91] and some in care home settings[92]. Some of our case study homes had developed their own systems, some used corporate systems, and some used 'off the peg systems'. Only one home used a computer-based model, which some staff found difficult at first and which was used in conjunction with paper-based information (for example, a paper copy of the plan retained in each resident's room).

One study home was developing its own more socially-oriented, dementia-specific care planning model. The model being developed avoided use of the word 'problem' and focused on strengths, needs and individual preferences. It had three core component plans: direct care, physical care and recreation/social care. It was also intended that it would include: a likes/dislikes checklist; a general health assessment form; a personal routines assessment; a dependency rating; a carers' strain rating; and possibly an assessment of the individual's ability to engage in activities.

Staff roles in care planning

In different homes, different people are responsible for compiling and updating care plans. There is no single 'right model'; it depends on staffing structures and management systems. Usually a senior staff member (senior care or primary nurse) has responsibility for the care plan and keyworkers and other staff contribute in different ways. It is most important that staff at all levels, but particularly the staff who deliver most personal care, are involved in care planning and have a sense that they 'own' the care plans. If this ownership does not develop, staff will not be committed to implementing the plans.

Consistency of care is very important for people with dementia. Good written care plans can help ensure consistency, but homes usually have a variety of other approaches to ensure consistency of care as staff come and go on shifts. For example, our study homes variously passed information from one shift to another through verbal handover meetings as well as 'communications books' and daily diaries. The effectiveness of such arrangements is as much a result of good management and teamwork as the detail of the system used[93].

The importance of the manager's role in ensuring that care plans are full, appropriate and implemented should not be underestimated:

> Managers conduct the process of care planning. It is their responsibility to see that an effective assessment is carried out, that objectives are defined, that action is agreed and implemented, that progress is reviewed, that full and accurate records are kept, that all other participants are properly involved, and that the resident's wishes are always paramount. In practice some of the details of these tasks ... may be delegated to another member of staff, but the manager always retains the responsibility for ensuring that they happen. (Coleman et al, 1999[94], p 37)

Some important points about care planning are summarised in Box 3.3.

Therapies and activities

Therapies

The range of therapies in use in dementia care has expanded, although for most therapies there is still limited research evidence about what is effective, for whom and in what circumstances[95]. Our study homes varied considerably in the extent to which they used 'therapies', including:

- aromatherapy[96]
- reflexology
- reminiscence[97]
- validation[98]
- Sonas[99]

Box 3.3: Some key points about care planning

Care planning should:
- address social relationships, sexuality, spirituality, mental health, activities and physical health
- reflect the individual resident's abilities, needs, preferences and biography
- include appropriate risk assessment and management
- address relationships with relatives
- address financial and legal issues
- produce up-to-date documents that staff use and find helpful
- include regular reviews
- allow changes to be introduced as and when required
- be undertaken by the staff who know the resident best, including unqualified care staff, care staff on different shifts and others who contribute to the individual's care
- involve the resident and their relatives as much as possible
- meet all statutory requirements
- include a record that is kept in the resident's room for staff and, where appropriate, relatives (see page 32) to read at any time
- be addressed in staff training
- be viewed as a team activity
- be a management priority.

- reality orientation (RO)[100]
- Snoezelen, or multi-sensory stimulation[101].

The therapies used in each home were determined by the home manager based on their views about the desirability and efficacy of particular therapies and on the interests and skills of staff. Managers rightly pointed out that it is important that staff have appropriate training before engaging in therapeutic activities. On the whole, managers and staff felt that these therapies were very useful additions to the home's repertoire of care but not essential for good practice.

Occupation and activities

It is important for the well-being of people with dementia that they have opportunities for occupation and involvement in the world around them. Yet we know that, in many care settings, people with dementia spend much of their time in an unoccupied and passive state[102]. Moreover, a care setting that gives an overall impression of a quality social and physical environment may nevertheless be providing low levels of engagement and well-being for individuals with dementia. We can understand this, and respond more appropriately to people with dementia, if we appreciate that it is often the immediate social and physical environment that matters more to people with dementia than the broader social milieu[102].

We should be clear that in advocating occupation and social engagement we are not advocating 'doing activities' in a simplistic way. Rather we are suggesting that homes need to develop imaginative approaches to occupation and activity[103].

Activities need to be tailored to the residents' individual interests, personalities and preferences at a particular time. Variety is important[104] and the range of activities that our study homes found useful are listed in Table 3.1. In several study homes the emphasis was on 'ordinary life' and on ensuring that residents had 'quality time' rather than organised group activities. Staff generally agreed that, as dementia becomes more advanced and concentration span shortens, it is more difficult to engage people. Activities need to be adjusted accordingly. In particular, as the dementia increases, sensory-based occupation and

Table 3.1: Useful activities with residents in dementia care homes

- Music and movement sessions
- Dancing
- Singsongs
- Weekly church services
- Quizzes
- Concerts
- Bingo
- Knitting bee
- Games such as draughts, skittles and darts
- Involvement in domestic tasks such as peeling potatoes, setting tables, dusting, making sandwiches, baking, handwashing clothes
- Art sessions such as painting
- Readings of poetry and local tales
- Weekly sherry party before Sunday lunch
- Barbecues
- Shopping from the 'weekly trolley'
- Using the 'bar' in the home
- Gardening or just spending time in the garden
- Having a car in the garden for people to sit in or tinker with
- Involvement in festivals and personal special occasions such as birthdays or anniversaries
- Individual and group outings, for example, to the seaside, circus, local garden centres, shopping, cafes, walks

occupation linked with everyday activities will become more appropriate[105]. Ideas about how to engage people with different levels of dementia have been advancing significantly and homes should ensure that their practice is informed by this recent work[106].

Occupation and activities including involvement in everyday activities need to be organised and this has implications for staffing that are discussed in Chapter 4.

Outings

Managers in a couple of our study homes reported that they were moving away from large group outings to more individual outings because they are more 'ordinary' and less stigmatising. However, staff sometimes resist this change because they like the 'big outings'. Whatever the size of the group, it is important that vehicles are not 'badged' in a way that stigmatises the occupants. It is also, for similar reasons, important that staff wear their own clothes rather than staff uniforms.

Homes identify two requirements for taking residents on outings: staff time and transport. The latter is less of a problem when homes are located in an area where it is possible to walk out to shops, local parks and so on. One study home demonstrated how we can extend the boundaries of what is possible. It very successfully took people with severe dementia on an outdoor adventure holiday organised with the Calvert Trust[107].

Pets

Observing and interacting with animals and birds can be rewarding for people with dementia. Only one of our study homes had a resident with their own pet – a bird which the resident kept in her own room. However, animals and birds featured in homes in a variety of other ways:

- bird tables, or, in one case, an aviary in the garden
- the home having a pet cat
- regular visits by the manager's dog or the neighbour's cat 'dropping in'
- regular visits by a 'Pat a Dog' (this is a scheme run by a charity to provide specially trained dogs to visit care homes and similar services).

On the whole, managers suggested that it was easier to have 'visiting pets' as they found it difficult to ensure that 'house pets' were properly cared for. One way to have visiting pets is to encourage relatives and friends to bring their pets along to the home.

Mealtimes and nutrition

People with dementia can easily become malnourished and dehydrated. As well as paying attention to nutritional needs, homes should pay attention to the social aspects of mealtimes[108].

Some key factors, identified in the literature[108] and our case studies, that are important in ensuring high quality mealtimes and good nutrition include:

- checking residents' weight regularly
- assessing each resident's fluid and food needs and monitoring intake
- ensuring good dental and oral health
- ensuring catering staff have the time, skills and motivation to find out about residents' likes and dislikes and to respond to them
- providing a choice of menus and assisting residents with dementia in being able to make a choice
- providing the option of a snack or 'finger food' if a resident refuses main meals
- providing flexible breakfast and supper times to suit individual residents
- ensuring food is of good quality, varied and well presented
- providing special food for celebrations
- welcoming relatives and friends to join meals
- ensuring a good dining environment (for example, with minimum distractions, with appropriate table layouts, with cues of appetising cooking aromas)
- avoiding the dining room being set up more than about 30 minutes before the meal
- making kitchen facilities available for relatives to use to make drinks and snack meals
- encouraging residents with dementia to assist with meals, for example, in preparing some food, in setting or clearing tables or washing up
- making mealtimes more of a social occasion by having staff eat with residents
- considering how best to arrange mealtimes to meet the needs of people who retain good social and manual skills as well as those who need more assistance
- ensuring that staff are trained in how best to assist people with dementia to eat.

Physical and mental health

Homes that specialise in dementia care must ensure that their focus on dementia does not lead to neglect of physical health needs. Managers must be confident that physical health problems will be identified and appropriately treated[109]. Since people with dementia may not be able to verbalise their pain or discomfort, staff need to be especially alert to the possibility of health problems. Treatment of the range of health problems that is likely to arise among residents with dementia requires homes to have good links with general and specialist health services (see

Chapter 2). Homes should, however, do more than this. They should endeavour to maintain and promote physical health for their residents through the well recognised principles of good diet, appropriate exercise, accident prevention and preventative care from chiropodists and dentists, for example.

It is particularly important that homes are alert to the fact that people with dementia can have other mental health problems. For example, over 50% of people with dementia in residential homes are depressed[110].

Managing medication

All care homes need to have sound policies and procedures for the storage and administration of medication. In dementia care homes, drugs are used for treating physical problems as well as mental health problems such as depression, anxiety, severe insomnia, agitation and psychotic symptoms. There is much variation in the levels of neuroleptic medication (also known as antipsychotics or major tranquillisers) used in dementia care facilities to manage residents' behaviour[111]. There are also concerns about inappropriate use of such medication[112]. The use of neuroleptics needs to be considered as part of a holistic care plan for each individual resident and in the context of overall management strategies to ensure high quality care[113]. Some of the recommendations that have been made[113] for good practice in dementia care are summarised below:

- Develop an overall approach to care that uses non-drug and drug treatments appropriately.
- Ensure the home has appropriate systems to record and review medication.
- Train staff in understanding non-medical and medical approaches to care, including the role of medication in handling difficult behaviour.
- Ensure staff are alert to the possible adverse effects of medication and the need to report any concerns.
- Discuss medication and its effects with relatives (subject to issues of consent and capacity).
- Make full use of the expertise available from GPs, nurses, consultants and pharmacists.
- Ensure the home's medication procedures comply with the law relating to consent.

Palliative care, death and dying

The management of palliative care, death and dying are all the more sensitive in dementia care when it can be difficult for staff to assess how people with dementia are feeling and what their needs are. Homes should ensure that they have access to palliative care expertise when necessary. They also need to consider how to ensure that person-centred care is maintained for people with dementia who are dying. There are several sources of advice for care homes generally[114] and some guidance specific to dementia care[115].

Working with relatives

Relatives' preferences about involvement after admission vary considerably, in part depending on the nature and quality of their past and current relationships with the person with dementia. The relationship between relatives and care homes is complex and often "characterised by tensions, misunderstandings, misperceptions and poor communication"[116]. When involvement is facilitated by the home, many relatives choose to remain actively involved, often providing direct assistance[117]. It is important that homes negotiate a level of involvement to suit individual relatives and residents with dementia[118].

A partnership in care

The first step in involving relatives is to make it clear to them that the home values them and the part that they play in the resident's life.

> The ideal to work for seems to be one of 'shared care', in which staff and relatives co-operate in care planning, deciding on issues of risk, and consulting in all times of change or crisis. (Kitwood et al, 1995[119], p 76)

All of the homes in our study had the policy of encouraging relatives to visit at any time. They used a variety of approaches to maintain contact with relatives and involve them as partners in care (see Box 3.3). This emphasis on partnership with relatives must, of course, be set alongside concern to respect the wishes and privacy of the resident with dementia. Homes need to consider

Box 3.4: Involving and supporting relatives

- Make it very clear to relatives that they are welcome in the home at any time and can spend as much time there as they want.
- Accept that relatives vary in the extent and type of involvement that they want.
- Recognise that some relatives find it practically difficult to maintain contact, for example, because of work, family commitments or transport problems. Respond flexibly, for example, by arranging volunteer drivers or maintaining telephone contact.
- Encourage relatives to help themselves to refreshments when they visit and to join residents for meals.
- Involve relatives in social events such as barbecues and invite them to join festival celebrations such as Christmas dinner.
- Enable relatives to join in religious services in the home.
- Make sleepover accommodation available.
- Provide a quiet and private space where relatives can meet the resident other than in their bedroom.
- Have a relatives' notice board with details of relevant organisations, events, complaints procedure and so on.
- Ensure relatives meet the keyworker when the resident moves into the home.
- Involve relatives in drawing up and reviewing care plans.
- Ensure the care plan is readily available for relatives to read.
- Have regular (for example, four- or six-weekly) meetings between relatives and the keyworker to discuss the resident's care.
- Empower relatives to provide such practical care as they wish – even when this is more time consuming for staff.
- Provide a support group for relatives and/or individual counselling/support sessions.
- Provide contact details for other support services, for example the Alzheimer's Society or Cruse.
- When the resident dies, give relatives time to grieve and do not rush them to clear the room.
- After the resident dies, welcome relatives who wish to come back to the home either for an occasional visit or as regular volunteers.

carefully residents' views about information sharing with relatives in order to ensure that appropriate confidentiality is maintained.

Support for relatives

It is good practice for care homes to support relatives as well as residents[120]. Support is important at the time of admission when relatives are dealing with complex emotions and practical difficulties. Even after the person with dementia has settled in, relatives may need support in visiting; for example, they may need advice about how to respond if the resident does not recognise them or if it is difficult to engage the resident in conversation. Relatives also need support in the time leading up to, and after, the resident dies.

Staff and managers in all of our study homes viewed support for relatives as an important function. Three study homes provided support groups for relatives in which they could share their experiences and support each other. In one home the group was organised by an assistant manager, who was a qualified counsellor, working with the home's chaplain. In the other homes senior staff led the groups. Although it has been suggested that all homes for people with dementia should have relatives'/carers' groups[121], it is possible to provide good support in other ways. For example, the manager in one study home pointed out that group support was available from other organisations in the area and that they therefore offered more individual support, and sometimes intensive counselling. Again, the study homes' approaches to supporting relatives are summarised in Box 3.4.

Community links

A commitment to person-centred care and providing as 'ordinary' a life as possible involves maintaining residents' links with the world outside the home. Thus, making a home 'part of the local community' brings direct social benefits for people with dementia[122]. It also supports the sort of open organisational culture that is important in maintaining good dementia care[123].

Community links are greatly affected by the location of the home (see Section Two). For example, one study home in a city centre location found it easy for staff to take residents shopping, to coffee shops and so on. In contrast, a home in a deprived, redevelopment area was more isolated from the world around it because of concerns about security and about local school children taunting residents. The challenge of community links here was focused on building better relationships with the local school.

All of the study homes had local clergy coming in to take services and sometimes to spend time with individual residents. One home had been 'adopted' by a local church. Local schools sometimes had contact with homes but usually this was limited to events such as 'carol singing'. One manager commented that, although it was good for residents to see children in the home, it could be distressing for some of the children. She suggested that it was sometimes better to involve the children of staff or residents' families since it was then easier to ensure appropriate support.

Residents' money

It should not be assumed that everyone with dementia in care homes is completely unable to manage their money and valuables; individual assessments should be undertaken to determine what is appropriate for each person. Residents may have relatives who take responsibility for managing their financial affairs but sometimes care homes are involved directly. People with dementia are particularly vulnerable to financial abuse both by homes and by relatives. Guidance on managing residents' money is available from a variety of sources and homes should ensure that they have policies and procedures in place to meet legal and good practice requirements[124].

Risk management

Care homes sometimes need to protect people with dementia from hazards and harm. However, if people with dementia are to have the best possible quality of life, they also need to be empowered to make full use of their retained abilities. This involves some risk taking. Homes therefore need to think in terms of an extended concept of risk, not just about hazards and protection. Managers and staff in our study homes talked in terms of aiming to strike a good balance between the protection of residents and the quality of life gains that come from taking some risks.

Different care organisations have different formal and informal approaches to the management of risk[125]. At a practical level, case study homes tackled some 'risks' differently. For example, all homes had locked 'front' doors and secure garden areas. Some, but not all, homes allowed residents free and unaccompanied access to secure gardens or courtyards. Some, but not all, homes allowed residents to 'help out' in unit kitchenettes. Several homes cited food and hygiene regulations as precluding residents from preparing food to be shared with others. Most homes placed the main kitchen 'out of bounds' to residents, but one set aside an area of the kitchen in which groups of residents could do some baking under staff supervision. Similarly, while in most homes the laundry was out of bounds to residents, one home was happy for residents to come in to help with folding clothes and so on.

None of our study homes used physical restraint. Good practice requires that restraint should only be used in very exceptional circumstances and that it should be tightly controlled by procedures to protect against abuse[126]. Managers, however, also need to protect against the informal ways in which the environment, care practices, culture and so on can effectively serve to restrain residents, even when this is not their intended purpose[127].

Practice guidance on risk management is available[128]. Drawing on a number of sources[129] and our case studies we summarise in Box 3.5 some important messages for managers.

> **Box 3.5: Effective risk management**
>
> Managers should:
> - develop a clear risk policy and procedures that address the need to take risks as well as to protect residents from harm
> - ensure that the policy is known to all concerned; accept that different people (people with dementia, relatives, staff, managers, proprietors, other agencies) have different views about acceptable risk and involve them in risk decision making
> - talk to relatives about accepting that some accidents will happen if the home allows people the freedom that enhances their quality of life
> - ensure that staff are appropriately trained
> - make decisions about risk on the basis of individual assessments
> - keep decisions about risk under review as the abilities of people with dementia change
> - develop a culture in which staff feel free to discuss risk issues knowing that mistakes will be treated as opportunities for learning rather than defensive blaming of individuals
> - recognise that a degree of risk taking is important not only for individual residents but also for practice development.

> **Box 3.6: Effective practice to combat abuse**
>
> Managers should:
> - combat ageism and stereotype assumptions about people with dementia
> - know about different forms of abuse and what to look for
> - be open to the possibility that their staff might abuse residents
> - recognise the potential for relatives to abuse residents after admission
> - develop a culture in which staff will tell managers if they are concerned about the conduct of colleagues
> - have clear abuse policies and procedures that are implemented and monitored
> - build discussion of abuse into staff supervision arrangements
> - ensure that staff training addresses abuse
> - be prepared to confront suspected abusers.

Abuse

Abuse occurs in care homes for older people, and people with dementia are particularly vulnerable. Abuse is most often thought of as staff providing inadequate care or physically, emotionally or psychologically mistreating residents. However, abuse can also involve financial, sexual, racial and spiritual maltreatment[130]. There are several sources of practice guidance[131]. Managers must recognise that much abuse is subtle and that they need to address it at an organisational level as well as at the level of individual interactions[132]. Important components of effective managerial practice have been identified in Box 3.6, from the literature[133] and our case studies.

Legal and ethical issues

It is beyond the scope of this guide to provide detailed advice on the many ethical and legal issues for homes providing care for people with dementia[134]. Here we highlight three points. First, managers need to ensure that the interests of residents are protected in a context in which they have impaired mental capacity and much less power than either relatives or staff. Second, managers need to consider how to strike appropriate balances between the promotion of autonomy for people with dementia and decisions made by others in the 'best interests' of people with dementia. Third, managers need to deal with different and sometimes conflicting interests between staff and residents, and between individual residents and the wider group. It can be useful in such circumstances to involve a range of people in decisions: residents, staff, relatives, other professionals and so on. But this carries the risk that the views and interests of the person with dementia may be lost in the process. Advocacy is increasingly being recognised as an important means of protecting the interests of people with dementia[135]. The initiative of one of our case study organisations in developing an advocacy policy and procedures is one that other homes would do well to consider. Negotiation, mediation and arbitration have also been suggested to be useful approaches in resolving conflicts of interests in dementia care homes[136].

4

Staffing matters

Introduction

Good staffing has a direct and positive impact on the well-being of people with dementia in care homes[137]. The importance of good staffing cannot be overestimated. As one manager put it:

"A home is only as good as its worst care assistant."

Nationally there needs to be substantial investment in the development of care staff[138]. This chapter addresses core issues that managers must tackle if they are to ensure that their professional, care and support staff provide good dementia care.

Staffing levels and skill mix

There is no clear consensus about ideal staff:resident ratios in dementia care units. In part this is because staffing ratios are not the only determinant of the quality of care. We must also take into account the needs of the resident group, care staff skills, the contribution of support staff (see page 37) and the quality of management.

The Alzheimer's Society[139] suggests that the care staff:resident ratio should be no poorer than 1:5 for day shifts and 1:8 for night shifts. A range on either side of this (1.4–1.7) has been suggested elsewhere[140]. There have been cautionary notes that better staff:resident ratios are only beneficial if staff roles are clearly defined within an overall culture of person-centred social care[141].

The care staffing levels of the homes in this study varied. Where homes had dementia care units, these units had a more generous staff:resident ratio than the rest of the home. The most common ratio in our study homes was around 1:4 (including qualified staff but not managers). This was the ratio in four homes (although in one of these homes that ratio was approximately 1:5 on the late shift). Only one home had a better ratio; with approximately 1:3 in the morning a little less generous in the afternoon. The homes with ratios less favourable than 1:4 included one home with a 1:5 ratio. In another home the ratio was 1:6 in the high dependency unit and 1:8 in another unit for people with dementia. However, this home additionally employed servery staff in each unit between 7.30am and 2pm to free care staff from work associated with providing meals. In some homes senior staff 'floated' between units to ensure that qualified staff cover was available to all residents.

The night staff:resident ratios in our case study homes varied from 1:6 to 1:12. The variation was in large part related to unit size. Homes with small units had to have a member of staff on each unit and also had to ensure appropriate supervision by qualified staff. This led to their having relatively fewer residents per staff member than homes with larger units. Homes with large units generally took advantage of the economy of scale that this offered and had more residents per member of night staff. In considering night staff ratios, it is important to take into account the extent to which night staff are expected to undertake administrative or domestic tasks (such as helping with laundry work).

Two homes had arrangements for allocating miscellaneous, but important, tasks in the home. In Home A there were 'captains' appointed for specific tasks like generally overseeing use of the garden, provision of newspapers and so on. The manager in Home D took this approach further in that every member of staff had an area of responsibility in the home with tasks matched carefully to ability. The managers thought these arrangements played an important part in giving staff a sense of responsibility for the home as a whole rather than just their own unit.

In study homes with poorer staff:resident ratios, care staff felt under more pressure to 'get through the work'[142] rather than spend 'quality time' with residents. Having said that, no matter what staffing level existed, staff generally commented that they would like more time for one-to-one work with residents.

Occupation and activity is very important for people with dementia (see Chapter 3). It has been suggested that residents in care homes experience a more appropriately structured day if there is a member of staff responsible for the organisation of the day and its activities[143]. Our study homes, and their parent organisations, used a range of staffing strategies to promote occupation and activities, including:

- funding staff training in activities
- designating a member of staff in each unit to have special responsibility for activities
- giving a senior care worker responsibility to coordinate staff skills in activity work
- arranging sessional input from a resource worker to provide ideas and information about activities
- employing a part-time activity coordinator.

While specialist advice and input was welcomed, our study home managers were not all convinced about the benefits of having an activity coordinator. Some home managers argued that having a coordinator tended to reinforce a perception of activities as being distinct and special; this ran counter to their emphasis on quality activity throughout the life of the home. When homes choose to have an activity coordinator, managers must be clear about the nature of the role and the type of skills required if they are to ensure the appointment of someone who can work creatively with people with dementia and the rest of the staff team.

Arrangements for staff cover

Most study homes had their own 'bank staff' who could be called upon as needed to provide cover for holidays, sick leave and so on. In one home, however, bank staff tended to disappear into permanent jobs elsewhere, so the manager generally relied instead on cover from within the staff group, especially from part-time staff doing extra hours. Homes varied in their use of agency staff to cover for sickness and holidays but generally avoided their use as much as possible. Managers found it expensive to use agency staff and they were concerned that bringing in temporary staff in this way was inconsistent with good quality care because these staff were not familiar with the home's philosophy, practices and residents.

Staffing for day care and respite services

The staff skills needed for respite and day care are different from those needed for long-term care[144]. It is, therefore, important that any dementia care home that provides respite or day care, has staff who are specifically trained for this work. The manager of one home with day care advised that it is better to have dual residential and day care staff contracts. This gives flexibility to cover sickness and it reduces the risk that day care staff lose out on staff development opportunities that are geared around residential staff.

Support service staff

Homes should not underestimate the contribution made by support service staff (domestic, catering, laundry, maintenance and administrative) to providing quality care and an environment that affirms that residents are valued people.

All case study homes had dedicated kitchen and domestic staff, and there were only two homes without dedicated laundry staff. Some, but not all, homes had a 'handyperson' who, in some cases, also looked after the garden; other homes used contractors for the garden. The effect of having skilled practical support readily available was evident in the standard of maintenance inside and outside our study homes. Homes also had administrative posts and some managers noted the growing importance of this role as

> **Box 4.1: Some key elements of good support services**
>
> - Staffing levels for domestic and laundry work should be sufficient to ensure that care staff are not taken away from resident care to cover these tasks.
> - Domestic staffing arrangements should allow for prompt cleaning up after incontinence accidents.
> - The perennial problems of residents losing clothing or having it damaged in the laundry can be solved; the key to success is having an adequate number of designated and well-motivated staff in an in-house laundry.
> - As well as general laundry duties, laundry staff should have responsibility for collecting and returning residents' personal items, for appropriate laundry of 'special care' clothing, and for ironing and mending.
> - Catering staff need to be flexible and interested in residents as well as being technically proficient.
> - Catering staff should receive training in how best to meet the nutritional needs of people with dementia.
> - Catering staff should have opportunities to find out about residents' preferences and to get feedback about residents' views of the food provided.
> - Readily available maintenance services are crucial in ensuring that the appearance of the building is well maintained at all times; this is particularly important in promptly putting right some of the minor decorative damage that is common in dementia care units.
> - Gardens need to be maintained by people who are skilled and interested in gardening and not just by general maintenance staff; the gardener should have access to specialist advice on gardens for people with dementia.
> - There should be adequate administrative support for the home's management.
> - There should be good telephone and front-door reception arrangements.

administration is becoming more complex. Administrators often also covered reception and managers commented that it was important to have reception arrangements that did not involve staff being pulled away from resident care to receive visitors.

Managers must ensure that support staff are valued members of the staff team. In one study home in particular, the valuing of support staff was evident in how they described their role and the obvious pride they took in their work. Some important elements of good support services are summarised in Box 4.1.

Using volunteers

Most of our case study homes had some experience of using volunteers. Two homes made substantial use of volunteers; in both cases this was supported by their parent organisation's policies. For example, one organisation had developed a 'Volunteers Charter' and 'Volunteers Role' leaflets setting out how volunteers should be treated, what they should expect and what their responsibilities are. A volunteer coordinator worked for three sessions per week in the home and supported around 13 volunteers who provided activities for residents and spent time with residents who had few family visitors.

Another home had around 29 active volunteers, with other people providing occasional support.

Volunteers in our study care homes included:

- relatives of residents
- relatives of deceased residents
- people from local churches
- people who had responded to advertisements for volunteers in the local press
- people from a local volunteer bureau or from local Alzheimer's Society or Age Concern groups
- work experience students
- community service volunteers.

Volunteers may be involved regularly or occasionally and in different ways including working with residents, helping with social events, gardening and fundraising. Box 4.2 sets out some advice about using volunteers.

Staffing matters

Box 4.2: Using volunteers

- Find out about volunteering in your area; it may be easier to attract volunteers in some areas than in others.
- Be prepared to invest in recruitment if you want volunteers to play a significant role in the home.
- Ask staff what volunteers could usefully do and when it is most useful to have them around.
- Plan how you will use volunteers, taking into account the needs of the home and the skills of the volunteers.
- Be clear about your expectations of volunteers and discuss these expectations with them.
- Recognise that it can be difficult for volunteers to know what to do in a dementia care setting.
- Match volunteers with tasks that fit with their interests and skills.
- Recognise that it can be difficult to involve volunteers in extensive one-to-one contact with residents with dementia.
- Provide volunteers with training and support if you want to sustain their interest and commitment.
- Make sure volunteers feel appreciated and say 'thank you', for example through social events.

Staff recruitment

"Staff recruitment is a key factor in success."
(Manager)

Managers in our study homes variously identified the following factors as impacting on the ability of homes to recruit good staff:

- a general shortage of RMNs, especially 'good RMNs' with experience of dementia care
- location in high employment areas where other types of work are available
- location in high employment areas where care workers can opt for agency work, with better pay rates and without the constraints of a contract
- accessibility of the home by public transport
- competition from substantial numbers of other homes in the area.

Some of the approaches that study home managers found useful in attracting good applicants are summarised in Box 4.3.

Selection

Selection involves assessing the suitability of the individual for the post. However, staff selection must also ensure a good balance of personal attributes, skills and experience in the staff group as a whole[145]. And it must ensure that there is sufficient diversity in the staff group (for example in age, gender, ethnic background) to match staff with residents' needs and to allow residents to have choice about who provides their personal care.

It is widely recognised that good quality care is dependent on care staff having positive attitudes[146]. Several managers in our study said

Box 4.3: Attracting good staff

- Use 'word of mouth', in particular through personal contacts with existing satisfied members of staff.
- Advertise in local press and other local outlets such as newsagents.
- Advertise in local JobCentres.
- Combine recruitment for several homes to allow for the use of large adverts and the organisation of recruitment days.
- Use job titles and job descriptions that people will understand and that give a clear indication of what the job involves.
- Develop innovative approaches to recruitment (for example, Home A replaced job descriptions with informal, lively 'day in the life of...' leaflets describing the typical work day for different staff).
- Ensure adverts will be attractive to a wide age range, men and women, and people from minority ethnic communities.
- Ensure adverts will attract well-motivated people who are new to care work as well as experienced care workers.

their approach to staff selection focused on people's values, attitudes and warmth of feeling, rather than their qualifications and past experience. They explained that after appointment they could work to enhance the individual's knowledge and skills but that basic values and attitudes are difficult to change[147]. For similar reasons, managers thought it was better to have someone with no experience, whom they could develop, rather than someone with inappropriate experience that would have to be 'unlearned'. They also pointed out that there can be as much of a problem with qualified staff having to 'unlearn' inappropriate practice as there is with unqualified staff.

Drawing on the literature[148] and our case studies, we list in Table 4.1 some important characteristics that managers should seek in appointing care staff.

Table 4.1: Important characteristics to seek in care staff

- High regard for, and positive liking of, residents
- Emotional maturity and ability to understand self and others
- Capacity for good relationships with colleagues
- Sincerity
- Caring and compassion
- Honesty
- Strength of character
- Physical fitness
- Good communication skills
- Sense of humour
- Ability to interpret non-verbal signs and behaviour
- Awareness of boundaries such as personal space
- Good observational skills
- Practical care skills
- Ability to plan and organise
- Awareness of group dynamics and able to work with groups
- Awareness of the environment and how it affects people.

Additionally, for supervisory staff:
- Ability to be supportive and encouraging
- Ability to inspire the confidence of others
- Ability sensitively to deal with, and if necessary confront, poor practice.

Selection procedures

Study homes used a range of selection processes that aimed to give the applicant the opportunity to develop a realistic picture of the job as well as giving the home the opportunity to assess the applicant's response to residents and the care environment. In all study homes the manager played a central role in staff selection; their expertise in this is therefore an essential prerequisite for obtaining a good staff group. Selection processes used in our case study homes included:

- a one-hour discussion with applicants followed by applicants spending one hour with residents
- an 'open day' followed by an interview later in the week (the open day was intended to help people self-select prior to interview, but the home suspected that JobCentre requirements meant that few people opted out prior to interview)
- an interview followed by a 13-week trial period as 'bank staff' before the applicant or the home made a commitment to an employment contract.

Staff induction

"Train from the word go." (Manager)

All study homes attached great importance to staff induction. Induction minimally covers all statutory requirements and internal operating policies and procedures. However, it is also more than that. Induction is a major opportunity to instil into new staff the culture and standards of the home. Study homes that were part of larger organisations were often given a framework for their induction programmes. For example, Home A had developed an attractive individual induction booklet for staff to record their progress and it also operated a 'buddy system' for new staff. Generally the parent organisations' induction programmes were not dementia-specific and homes had to supplement them with their own approaches to introducing staff to more specific aspects of dementia care. Advice from our study homes is contained in Box 4.5.

Staffing matters

> **Box 4.5: Some advice about staff induction**
>
> - Do not overemphasise the 'knowledge' input; keep a strong focus on practice.
> - Ensure a strong emphasis on the philosophy and culture of the home.
> - Introduce key principles of person-centred dementia care.
> - Ensure a strong emphasis on teamworking.
> - Use existing trained staff to support new staff, for example through 'buddy' arrangements.

Since homes inevitably have some turnover of staff, induction training needs to be provided as an ongoing feature of the work of the home.

Staff retention

Staff turnover is not entirely negative. It contributes to bringing new ideas into the home and so counters institutionalising tendencies. Sometimes staff turnover indicates that a home is providing good foundation experience for people who then go on to further training in the caring professions. Turnover can, however, also have negative impact on quality of care. Some study homes had a very stable staff group, some had a stable core staff alongside a throughput of short-term staff and some had 'a retention problem' with substantial numbers of staff staying for a limited time. The following factors contribute to good levels of staff retention:

- lack of competition from other homes or other employment opportunities
- good initial selection (see pages 39-40)
- good induction and support for staff while they 'find their feet' in a new setting (see page 40)
- a good match between the reality of the work and the expectations of new appointees
- high staff morale and work satisfaction (see below)
- good team spirit
- a management style that fosters a sense of belonging and commitment
- good terms and conditions (see page 42-3)
- a sympathetic approach to staff personal circumstances (for example in arranging leave and rotas)
- good ongoing staff support, training and development (see pages 44-6).

Staff work satisfaction

Low staff satisfaction with their work is associated with higher rates of sickness and absenteeism. High staff satisfaction with their work is important for staff themselves and in ensuring good resident care.

Staff in our study homes often expressed pride in their work and clearly had a strong sense of commitment to 'doing things well'. This was reflected, in several homes, in staff undertaking 'extra' activities on an unpaid basis 'in their own time'[149]. Most staff said that they got considerable satisfaction from their work. Factors identified in the literature[150] and our case studies as contributing to staff satisfaction include:

- a friendly, relaxed atmosphere
- having time to get to know and work with residents individually
- being able to meet residents' needs
- good staffing levels
- knowing that when feeling stressed or struggling to cope, support will be available from colleagues
- good leadership
- management recognising the difficulties experienced by staff
- good staff support and supervision
- good, and particularly fair, levels of pay
- good conditions of service, such as shift patterns
- the possibility of career progression
- recognition of staff skills and experience
- clear role definition
- opportunities for staff to use their ideas and initiative
- good social relations in the home
- physical environment that facilitates good care (see Section Two)
- good staff facilities such as a pleasant staff room (see Section Two)
- a feeling of ownership
- being part of a team

- a sense of achievement and accomplishment
- approachable management
- managers who listen to staff and understand their difficulties
- opportunities for training and development.

Staff dissatisfactions were usually about conditions that they thought were unfair or demands they felt unreasonable. For example, staff in one home felt dissatisfied that conditions of service and pay rates were too low for the levels of responsibility they carried. Having said that, many staff stressed that, in practice, they set such complaints to one side because "we're not here for the money, we're here for the residents". In another home, staff dissatisfaction was expressed about high levels of sickness and staff turnover leading to extra demands on those who stayed. It was clear from our discussions that staff dissatisfaction could also rise if changes in the management of the home, or of individual units, created uncertainty or inconsistent expectations for staff.

Staff vary in how they experience working with people with dementia compared with working with other groups of residents. Their views are in part linked to the residents' levels of dementia. Some staff found working with people with dementia less physically tiring than working with other groups which involved more lifting and handling. Some staff found work with people with dementia less depressing than working with physically disabled residents; they pointed out that cognitively able residents could be very assertive and difficult. Some staff felt people with dementia were difficult to work with but they welcomed the challenge. These differences demonstrate that staff are as individual as residents. It is, therefore, as important to have person-centred staff management as person-centred resident care.

Valuing staff

Valuing staff must be an integral part of all of the home's policies, procedures and practices. However, staff and managers in our case studies mentioned some of the 'small things' that are important in conveying to staff that they are valued. These included:

- allowing staff to take 5 or 10 minutes 'time out' at any time when they feel they really need a break, and trusting them not to abuse this
- being flexible about rotas to try to accommodate staff personal needs
- sending a letter to staff acknowledging any incident of violence (this was much appreciated by staff)
- giving praise, thanks and tokens such as chocolates or flowers for special occasions or achievements.

Pay and conditions of service

Pay rates

We noted above that most staff describe their main motivation as 'caring' rather than financial reward[151]. However, pay rates are nonetheless important to staff and therefore indirectly affect the quality of care provided. It is not so much the absolute level of pay that matters to staff as whether they see their pay rates as being fair and reasonable for the work they do and in comparison with others[152].

Staff costs are a major factor in determining the financial viability of any home. One manager described the dilemma that arises when a home has to operate with a fixed budget. Should the manager go for lower wages, which brings the option of more staff? Alternatively, should the manager choose to have fewer but better rewarded staff who are more likely to stay and provide good quality care? Homes in this study generally reported having pay rates for care staff that were above the 'going rate' in the private sector but were generally slightly lower than local authority or NHS pay rates. The one private sector home in the study paid 'minimum wage' rates for care staff and staff generally felt that this undervalued them. The rates for staff employed as nurses were generally in line with NHS rates although one home exceeded this. One organisation in the study operated a bonus scheme for staff to 'share in any surplus'. Managers saw this scheme as being a way of involving staff and increasing their sense of ownership of the organisation.

Conditions of service

With the exception of the private sector home in the study, homes offered pension options and provided sick pay related to length of service. However, the generosity of sick pay schemes varied quite considerably. One organisation provided private health cover for staff. Managers knew that staff tended to say that they would prefer to have 'the money in their pocket' rather than private health cover; however, they found that staff were very appreciative of the cover when they needed to use it. Another organisation took a very firm line on sickness absence and used both 'sticks and carrots' to manage it. Perfect attendance for a year was rewarded with a £50 bonus. Alongside this was strict application of disciplinary procedures, and ultimately dismissal, for repeated sickness absences.

Managers were beginning to anticipate the potential impact of new requirements for parental leave and dependants' leave. Although such leave is unpaid it could potentially have a big impact for small organisations in managing the disruption in staffing.

In relation to conditions of service, one factor was very much appreciated by staff: having the organisation pay for their training. The opposite also applied: staff who do not receive financial support for training and development perceive this as an indication that they are not properly valued.

Shift patterns

Shift patterns varied for different staff grades within homes. There was also substantial variation between homes in their shift patterns. For example, the shift lengths of care staff varied from 7.5 hours (including a paid meal break) to 12 hours (with unpaid meal breaks), and the maximum number of days care staff worked without a break ranged from four days to seven days. In most homes, staff had a full weekend off duty every second or third week, but one home had a more complicated four-weekly rota involving one weekend on, one weekend off and two weekends of working one day.

Good dementia care must be founded on continuity and knowing the person with dementia. This has implications for how shifts should be organised. As well as addressing the needs of residents, shifts and rotas need to take account of the needs and preferences of staff. It is important to recognise that these vary. We found that some staff experienced long shifts (for example of 12 hours) as being too tiring and stressful. Similarly some disliked working seven days without a break. Others, however, found long shifts acceptable if this was accompanied by having longer breaks, for example of four days. Box 4.6 summarises some important points for managers in drawing up shifts and rotas in dementia care.

Box 4.6: Features of good staff shifts and rotas in dementia care

- Aim to ensure there is someone on each shift who knows each resident well.
- Promote continuity of care by building in time for communication in handovers.
- Ensure that full-time and part-time staff are involved in handover communication.
- Ensure that the evening shift runs late enough so that there is no pressure on staff to get residents to bed before they choose to retire.
- Avoid the 'them and us' of different staff teams; for example by having staff doing a mix of early and late shifts and by facilitating communication between day and night staff.
- Ensure that shift patterns build in appropriate staff rest and recuperation from the emotional and physical demands of dementia care.
- Ensure as much flexibility as possible in shift patterns to fit the preferences and circumstances of different staff members.

Table 4.9: Staff views about work attire

Uniforms	No uniforms
• nurses like them as a symbol of status • it helps residents to recognise staff • it helps relatives to recognise different grades of staff • it protects staff's own clothes	• 'it is more me than a trained nurse' • it feels more relaxed • 'it helps relatives see us as human beings' • protective clothing can be worn as and when necessary for the task

Staff uniforms

One interesting difference between our study homes was in whether or not staff wore uniforms. Where there were staff uniforms, there was often a distinction between different grades of staff (home managers never wore uniforms). Opinions differed about the merits of uniforms. The reasons staff and managers gave for and against uniforms are listed in Table 4.9.

It is important to note that 'uniforms' vary enormously in style and the image that they convey. For example, one organisation used quite traditional 'nurses uniforms'. Another organisation used overalls in a variety of styles but with the same print pattern; staff were pleased that "it is not clinical like a nurse's uniform". One device found to be particularly useful in aiding residents' recognition of staff was to have the staff member's personal name sewn on their overall.

Staff development

Investment in ongoing training and development is important for all grades of staff[153], and recent government initiatives[154] require the care home sector to pay more attention to staff training and development.

There are two main reasons why dementia care homes need to invest in staff development. First, there is a consensus that it is important to recognise and value the knowledge and contribution of care workers and to respond to their needs and difficulties[155]. Staff development programmes make a contribution to this. Second, staff training and support are essential factors in ensuring quality of long-term care for people with dementia[156].

Training

Commitment to staff training was an important factor in all homes in our study. Parent provider organisations generally had a strategic approach to staff training and, in some organisations, the home had a training budget devolved to the manager. Some larger parent organisations provided programmes of short courses available to staff in their various homes.

Several homes encouraged staff to do courses in care work provided by local colleges. Additionally, homes, both nursing and residential, used local community-based professionals to provide training sessions and advice and support for staff. However, it was sometimes the home managers who themselves provided much of the basic staff training. One organisation was setting up a 'training for trainers' programme to support managers in doing this. Homes with nursing staff tended to use nurses to train other care staff. This training partly involved informal and individual role modelling and advice. In some homes this type of approach was supplemented with regular short, for example 30-minute, training sessions provided by qualified staff and open to all staff. In one home some nursing staff were doing the ENB (English National Board) nurse teacher course.

Managers in the case study organisations varied in their views about NVQ/SVQs (National/Scottish Vocational Qualifications) and their general concerns are well recognised[157]. Several mentioned more specifically that these schemes are limited in the extent to which they meet the needs of dementia care settings. One home manager pointed out that it takes time to set up NVQ training in a new home. Managers also mentioned that it can be difficult for staff, particularly full-time staff, to find time for NVQ/SVQ work when they are coping with the demands of dementia care work. One manager was concerned that assessment in NVQs is very dependent on the individual assessors.

Despite the above reservations, several organisations were very committed to NVQs/SVQs and encouraged staff to pursue these qualifications, sometimes to level 3 or 4. For example, one organisation aimed to get a high proportion of its staff NVQ qualified and it had set up a coaching scheme to support this. It also offered a lump sum financial reward to individual staff who completed an NVQ.

Dementia-specific training

One of the major issues for specialist dementia care homes is how best to provide specific training in dementia care. Such specialist dementia training is important if staff are to understand what it is like to be a person with dementia and how they can best respond in person-centred ways. Organisations sometimes 'buy in' specialist dementia training and sometimes develop their own in-house programmes. In either case they should consider carefully how any programme will fit the specific needs of their service and organisation[158]. They should also ensure that the training is student-centred and builds on the experiences of individual members of staff[159].

The approaches adopted in our case studies included providers:

- supporting groups of staff to complete the Alzheimer's Society's 'Care to Make a Difference' training programme
- developing a two-day in-house 'understanding dementia' course which was first rolled out to home managers and unit managers, and subsequently to all staff working with people with dementia
- working with a local Dementia Services Development Centre to implement and evaluate dementia training programmes across a number of its homes
- encouraging staff with NVQ2 to complete a 'Dementia Workbook' under the guidance of a mentor; successful completion carried 200 CATS points and the award of a certificate by the organisation (the 'Dementia Workbook' included modules on the nature of dementia and managing specific problems; individual care; activities; communication; and an 'open learning' case study)
- enabling individual members of staff to undertake training in dementia-specific therapies such as Sonas or tools such as dementia care mapping (DCM).

Overall, our home managers attached more importance to all staff having good foundation training in dementia care than to some staff developing skills in more specific therapeutic techniques.

Broader approaches to staff development

Training is important but it will not in itself ensure good dementia care. Training needs to be part of a staff development strategy linked with broader management approaches to promoting a positive culture of care[160]. Homes should have systematic ways of identifying staff skills and experiences, and of considering their development needs. Homes should adopt a range of approaches to meet staff development needs. Some ideas for doing this are described in Box 4.7.

Box 4.7: Some ideas for staff development

- Be imaginative about staff development and do not restrict it to formal training.
- Remember that trained staff need updating with the latest practice ideas.
- Use any opportunities for practitioners in local services to provide advice, coaching or training.
- Establish a system of staff appraisals that includes the identification of development needs.
- Empower staff to take control of their personal development; for example, one organisation allowed some grades of staff £250 to use for personal development.
- Pay attention to the development needs of support service staff.
- Develop one-to-one 'coaching' by more skilled and experienced staff.
- Provide opportunities for staff to gain experience of working in different units with residents with different needs and colleagues with different skills.
- Create a culture in which staff achievements are recognised and valued; for example, one of our case study homes covered the walls of the staff room with staff certificates.
- Consider financial rewards for staff achievements; for example, one organisation offered a lump sum financial reward to staff for completion of an NVQ.
- Ensure as far as possible that the staffing structure makes career progression an option for staff; for example, avoid gaps in 'the ladder' of staff grades being so big that promotion is virtually impossible.

Section Two:
Designing dementia care homes

5 Design principles and processes

Introduction

A successful home is the product of several factors, only one of which is good design. Other factors, related to good quality care, staffing and management, are discussed in Section One. The success of a home is measured in a number of ways, but primarily by the well-being of the residents, which is related to the quality and commitment of the staff and management. Commercial success, in the form of financial viability, is also important. It is ultimately measured by the bottom line of the annual accounts but is routinely measured by occupancy. Good and pertinent design will provide the platform on which these other success factors can be based.

Care home design must take account of regulatory issues related to town planning, building control, fire regulations, health and safety, disability discrimination, environmental health, national minimum standards, and registration and inspection. They are not covered specifically in this document, as interpretation may vary according to local circumstances. Similarly, fundamental aspects regarded as standard good practice in the design of care homes have been covered in many publications[161] and are not considered here. This chapter begins by outlining the principles of good design before describing the processes by which good design is produced and translated into practice.

Principles and features of good design

The basic accommodation needs of people with dementia are no different from those of the rest of society. People with dementia need security, safety and comfort in a pleasant and stimulating environment. However, for people with dementia there are additional requirements, which reflect their dependency needs, resulting from impaired memory, learning and reasoning processes.

In the context of design, dementia should be regarded as a disability, and the aim should be to produce a therapeutic design and environment to barrier-free standards. It is often said that there is no single right way to design a care home. This is particularly true of homes designed for people with dementia because of the wide range of dependency and care needs. However, there is consensus about the important principles and features that should to be taken into account when designing for people with dementia.

There are two ways of summarising the international consensus. One is agreement on principles, the other agreement on design features.

The consensus on principles of design includes:

- design should compensate for disability
- design should maximise independence
- design should enhance self-esteem and confidence
- design should demonstrate care for staff
- design should be orientating and understandable
- design should reinforce personal identity
- design should welcome relatives and the local community
- design should allow control of stimuli.

The consensus on design features includes:

- small size
- familiar, domestic, homely in style
- plenty of scope for ordinary activities (unit kitchens, washing lines, garden sheds)
- unobtrusive concern for safety
- different rooms for different functions
- age-appropriate furniture and fittings
- safe outside space
- single rooms big enough for lots of personal belongings
- good signage and multiple cues where possible, for example, sight, smell, sound
- use of objects rather than colour for orientation
- enhancement of visual access
- controlled stimuli, especially noise.
(Marshall, 1998, p 12[162])

These lists are not necessarily exhaustive but they summarise clearly the most important issues to be considered by the designer confronting the challenge of designing for people with dementia.

In addition, from a commercial viewpoint, good design:

- results in greater staff efficiency
- creates more opportunity for well-being in residents
- attracts family decision makers
- attracts purchasers
- can improve occupancy rate and therefore sustain income
- should provide flexibility – possibly for alternative use
- results in cost-effective use of space
- minimises maintenance costs.

The design brief

A care home for dementia is intended primarily for people whose memory, learning and reasoning processes are impaired, and who may experience high levels of stress in their normal daily lives.

The decision to consider building such a care home should be based on identified needs supported by market research. This should include study of demographic trends and consultation with the appropriate referral agencies within the local healthcare sector, the availability of suitably qualified staff and the sure knowledge of confirmed and continuing demand within the specified catchment area[163]. In particular, the relevant registration authorities should be consulted at an early stage.

The selection of a suitable site will usually be the responsibility of the provider and the eventual choice will depend on the primary factors of availability, site area, topography, access and location in a community setting. Realistically, the overriding factor will be 'availability' and may be dictated by circumstances, for example, a site already in ownership, a redevelopment opportunity, replacement on the site of an existing home or simply the only site available in the area.

The composition and responsibilities of the project group assembled to agree the brief and progress the pre-contract stages will vary depending on the size and structure of the organisation. Larger organisations will be able to assemble a two-tier system – a design team in addition to a project group. In smaller organisations, all responsibilities may be handled by one group – the owner and the architect. In the latter case, it is even more important that sound advice is sought to ensure that the actual requirements of the provider are translated satisfactorily into the ultimate design and specification.

At the outset the designer should be provided with a budget for the building based on the site value, the client's income and expenditure projections, and the financial arrangements for funding the development. The degree of flexibility required in design to allow for possible future alternative uses should also be agreed.

Inevitably there will need to be compromise in design, either because of financial constraint or conflict of opinion between architect and care practitioner. A successful outcome will emerge only if there is consensus within the project group, which is written into the design brief. All parties have a responsibility to commit to the brief and the parameters of variation within the budget should be clear to the designer.

In addition, there will need to be compromise when faced with the varied care needs of residents because of the potential range of dependency. It is also probable that future residents will be more frail on entry; they may require more cueing features and perhaps more advanced technological facilities.

The challenge, therefore, is to produce a design that is both innovative and sensitive, and capable of allowing the creation of a homely atmosphere in which residents can enjoy living, perhaps as a home for life. It is therefore even more important that architects familiarise themselves with the nature of physical and mental impairments and the environmental needs of people with dementia. When designing for people with dementia, emphasis must also be placed on the opportunity for residents to live with dignity and to maintain or enhance self-esteem.

The building will fulfil two primary purposes – as a home for the residents and, of equal importance, as a workplace for staff. Therefore, the designer's objective is to provide an environment in which these two primary purposes can be achieved and good quality care can be provided economically and efficiently.

In most cases the architects for the case study homes succeeded in designing buildings that took into account their clients' special needs. In this context 'the client' is multifaceted:

- company management – 'the owner' (responsible for instructing, briefing, paying the bills)
- operational staff and managers (who provide care)
- building management staff (responsible for design and maintenance)
- the purchaser of care home places, including social services, health services, relatives and self-funding individuals.

Architects are therefore responsible for translating the requirements of this multi-client group into a workable design. There may be difficulties that arise from the varied and sometimes conflicting wishes of the respective elements of 'the client', even though in some instances detailed design briefs are available or a tried and tested design is replicated. In other situations the design brief may be developed with the architect. When the client is uncertain, the choice of architect (or design advisor with relevant experience) is even more crucial.

Whether an architect or a design and build contractor (see below) is appointed, the provider must be satisfied that they are capable of producing a home that meets the provider's requirements, on time and within budget. References should be obtained, previous clients contacted, and care homes for which they have been responsible visited with the architect or the contractor. It is also important to ensure that the architect has specific experience of designing for people with dementia. The provider must at the least be satisfied that the architects are capable of finding out what living in and operating a home caring for people with dementia is really like before the design brief and the specification are finalised. Above all, the provider must be satisfied that their wishes, as expressed in the brief, are recorded correctly, and that each element satisfies a 'value for money' examination.

The pitfalls that can leave the provider disappointed include:

- inadequate design brief
- inadequate specification
- inexperienced architect or design and build contractor
- inexperienced mechanical and electrical (M&E) consultant (the cost of the M&E element can represent 30% of the contract value).

Procurement methods

The decision on which procurement route to follow needs to be made at an early stage. In addition to the conventional route involving the appointment of an architect, specialist advisers and builders selected by competitive tender, there are several alternatives including 'design and build'. This method is being used increasingly to reduce the overall project timescale, to identify and control costs from an early stage and to significantly advance the date of occupation. By coincidence, a design and build approach was utilised for five of the homes visited. Such routes, however, require careful monitoring by the provider, or their advisor, to ensure that the design and specification meet their requirements and that the contract value is within budget.

> Whatever the procurement route, one piece of unexpected information that the provider does not wish to hear is that the final cost is going to exceed the agreed budget!

In addition to the above, it is important that the architect and the contractor fully understand the need to complete all minor defect or maintenance items *before* the handover. The move to a new home is stressful enough for residents without further distress when work continues after occupation.

Managing the project

The opening of a new home should be treated as a special project on its own – not just the building contract but also the operation of setting up and opening the home. This is particularly so when the residents will be an existing group of residents who have to move from homes or hospitals scheduled for closure. The transfer time, depending on numbers, is much shorter than when group transfer is not involved. A liaison officer should be appointed:

- to work with the building contract management and the operational management to ensure that completion and handover dates are monitored
- to arrange a familiarisation programme for the person ultimately responsible for the maintenance of the building and for training in the use and operation of all relevant equipment
- to arrange for the selection, procurement and delivery timetable of furniture and household goods and setting up new orders with existing and/or new suppliers.

The design process: key messages

Some of the most important points about ensuring the successful and smooth implementation of good design are summarised in Box 5.1.

Box 5.1: Making good dementia care design happen

- Ensure that the role of the project team is clearly defined and members are carefully selected, but keep the numbers to a minimum to improve communication and decision making.
- Allow adequate time for site acquisition, planning and building.
- Make sure that the brief and schedule of accommodation are complete.
- Check thoroughly at the outset to ensure that the architect has relevant knowledge and experience – this will save time and money and will improve the prospects of achieving an effective and efficient design.
- Allow adequate time for the negotiation of contracts and fees and agree all terms before signing building contracts.
- Double check the specification and quantities for household items.
- Allow adequate time for post-contract processes – check with other providers if necessary.
- Before interior decoration commences, appoint a liaison officer with a clear brief and authority to link the building contract with the 'setting up home' project.
- Allow realistic time to reach full occupation.
- Pay close attention to detail in design and specification – this can enhance the quality of life for people with dementia.

6

Design in practice

Introduction

This chapter describes the design of each of our case study homes. The homes visited were located in urban or suburban settings with sites of varying shape, size and contours. For each home the background and approach to design is described and, in addition, outline ground-floor plans demonstrate the design approach.

Based on our observations and discussions with staff and managers, we highlight the features that either enhance the home *or* have a limiting influence on the success of the home. We also include comments, where offered, from groups of staff, management and relatives to illustrate their views about the buildings and their facilities. Full details of space provision, accommodation and capital costs are provided in the Appendix. This chapter concludes with a summary of common issues highlighted by the case studies.

Home A

This home was located in an urban setting and provided care for 36 older people with dementia. It was completed in early 1993 to replace a wing of an adjacent hospital, scheduled for closure. The provider was registered as a charitable trust.

The need for care for older people with dementia in the area was established by the former health authority and was essentially demand-led. There were people out of town in need of care whom the authority wanted to locate in a more central position and in specialist accommodation. No formal research was undertaken, the forecast for future need being provided by the health authority and social services from in-house evidence.

Pressure was exerted by the health authority to complete and commission the home before April 1993 – the implementation date for the Community Care Act – which imposed tight deadlines. The authority provided a 100% grant to build the home and retained the freehold, while the charitable trust held a long lease. In addition, the trust received an annual grant towards running costs from the authority.

At the outset a small project group was formed, including the director of nursing of the charitable trust and a representative from the former health authority. As a standard design brief already existed, the group's task was to adapt the brief to meet needs identified by the authorities and the constraints of the site.

The only site readily available adjoined an existing trust home for frail older people, and was owned by the authority. It was smaller than ideally required and resulted in a two-storey design.

The trust had already established a policy of adopting a group-living approach for care homes. However, subsequent operational experience had led them to believe that groups of 12/13 people were too large for dementia care and that groups of eight or nine and a staff to resident ratio of around 1:4 were more appropriate. As the health authority requirement was for a specific number of places (36), the design was based on four groups of nine.

Mainly because of the contractual relationship and financial arrangements with the health authority, the home was registered as a nursing home.

Home A Plan: Ground floor

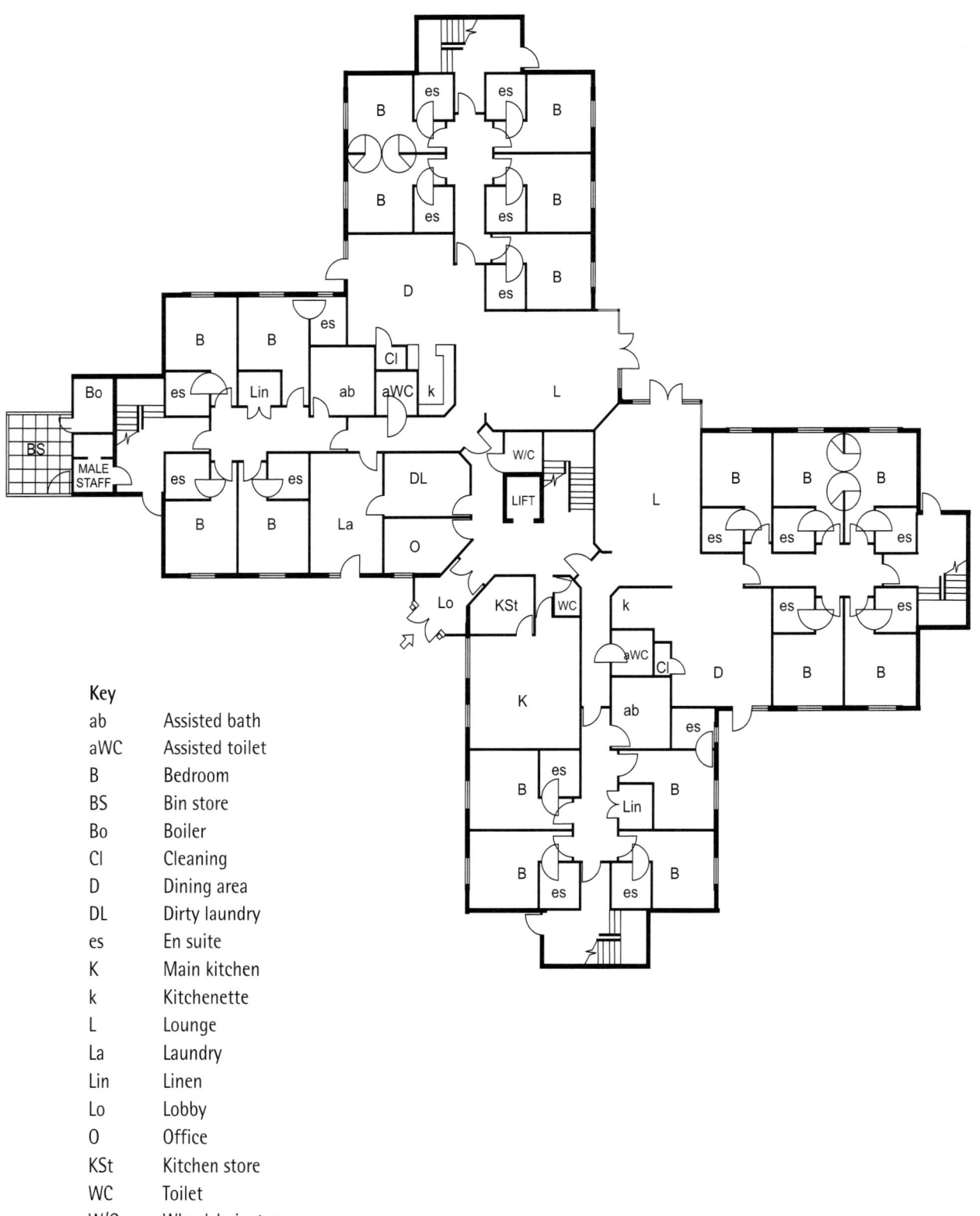

Key
- ab — Assisted bath
- aWC — Assisted toilet
- B — Bedroom
- BS — Bin store
- Bo — Boiler
- Cl — Cleaning
- D — Dining area
- DL — Dirty laundry
- es — En suite
- K — Main kitchen
- k — Kitchenette
- L — Lounge
- La — Laundry
- Lin — Linen
- Lo — Lobby
- O — Office
- KSt — Kitchen store
- WC — Toilet
- W/C — Wheelchair store

Design and use of building

The care home was purpose-designed as a home for older people with dementia (Home A Plan). It was built in 10 months within budget, using a design and build contractor.

The design was based on a cruciform plan form on two floors with nine residents' rooms in each group, arranged in clusters of four and five at the end of each leg of the cruciform. Four pairs of rooms could be linked to create accommodation for couples. All day rooms on the ground floor had direct access to terraces in the gardens. Unusually for a home built in 1993, showers were incorporated in en suites.

Separate lounge and dining areas, located in the internal angles of the cruciform, served each group – an arrangement which effectively separated sleeping and living zones and shortened the corridors. Although these areas straddled the corridor, they were not compartmentalised and had generous openings to the corridor, allowing easy transfer and the opportunity for joint use on special occasions. (This arrangement is not always possible as some fire officers insist on the physical separation of corridors and adjoining rooms.) There was no quiet room.

Small kitchen areas located near the dining rooms were used only by staff for making hot drinks and dishwashing. Main meals were distributed to all residents in heated trolleys from the central kitchen.

Safe wandering routes, intended as a special feature, relied on the residents using stairs at the end of each leg of the cruciform and involved the use of both floors. However, as a consequence of two residents falling on the stairs, secondary high-level baffle handles were fitted to the doors leading to the stairs. This curtailed the wandering routes and essentially created 'dead end' corridors, which appeared to cause some distress. Notwithstanding this, it is the home's policy to "give access to anyone who wants to use the stairs at any time". Free access to the gardens had also been limited to use only with staff supervision.

Snoezelen facilities – a moderate success – had been introduced in the former hairdressing room and although the loss of the latter was regretted, a similar facility existed in the home immediately next door and most residents enjoyed making a special visit to the hairdresser.

An old car, a shed and a greenhouse brought familiarity to the grounds and attracted residents, but footpaths were not continuous and therefore not ideal. Soft landscaped areas set out in isolated beds could have been improved by being linked.

Photograph 1: A free-standing seat would be more useful than the over-large drop-down seat, and a low-level screen more helper-friendly

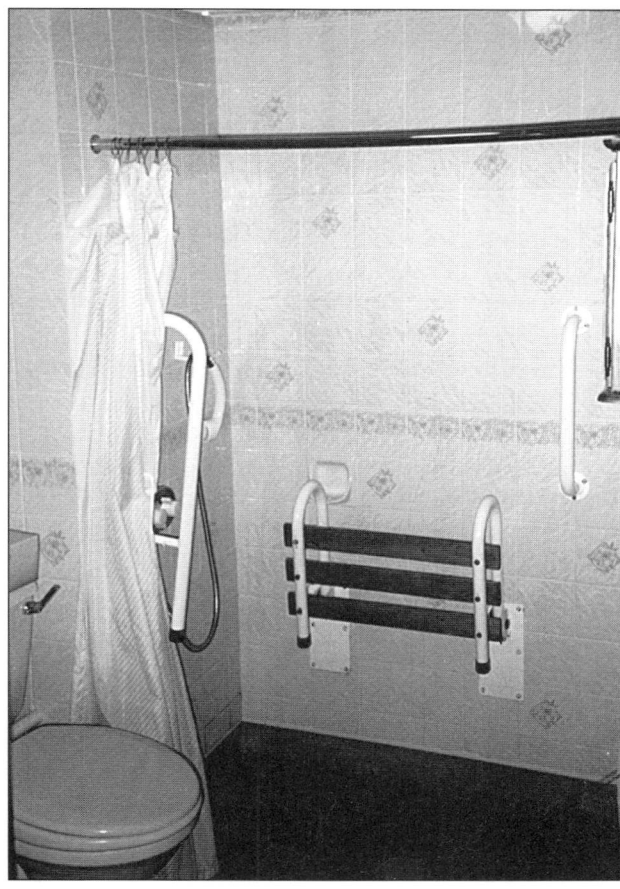

Box 6.1: Design features – Home A

Enhancing features
- group sizes and the arrangement of residents' rooms at the end of the cruciform legs, separating the group accommodation neatly into sleeping and daily living areas
- general attention to detail such as residents' room doors which were lockable from the inside but which could be opened in an emergency from the outside, giving the residents a sense of ownership and security
- free swing door closers on residents' room doors
- shower controls outside the showering zone
- Snoezelen room
- textured paint finish on corridor walls, coupled with the use of a dado rail, creating an attractive durable finish to replace wallpaper and borders which had been damaged by inquisitive residents.

Limiting features
- under-provision of staff facilities – lockers had to be located in laundry
- lack of protection for staff when assisting residents in the shower; the shower curtains were a hindrance when assistance was being provided (see Photograph 1)
- fixed showerhead in en suites – a variable head position with a flexible hose would be preferable
- pre-determined bed positions – in several rooms it was observed that neither of the two optional positions was used – this created minor problems related to the location of room service socket outlets
- the WC in the en suite bathroom was not in view from bed positions
- wandering routes limited to one floor because of 'baffled' doors at the ends of short corridors
- the kitchenette adjoining the dining area was not used by residents; it could have been more user-friendly, an up-stand on the 'customer' side created a psychological barrier
- the problem of disturbing noise transfer between group lounge and dining room; no quiet space available other than the Snoezelen room.

Home B

The provider – a major national charity – opened its first specialist dementia care home in 1989. It decided to extend the number of such homes after investigating need across the country. This decision was based on the increasing incidence of dementia within its numerous residential care homes. Research involved canvassing local authorities and examining care policies and generated arrangements with two authorities. Based on this research a further home was opened in 1996 and the case study home was opened in 1997.

The initial enthusiastic response from the second local authority diminished as unitary authority status approached. Senior members of staff who had been involved in negotiations moved on, the political environment changed and the offer of enhanced fees, to reflect the 'extra care' needed by people with dementia, was reduced drastically. When the home opened there was virtually no recognition of the cost of specialised care and costs were subsidised by the charity. Eventually, the operational balance sheet of the home was partly redressed by other authorities prepared to reflect the true cost of dementia care in their fees.

The policy of the provider organisation was to provide dementia care in residential homes, ideally in single-storey buildings with emphasis on easy access to the gardens. It was also acknowledged that people with dementia needed more day space than residents in a standard care home, that they benefited from living in smaller groups, and that the welfare of staff was as important as the welfare of residents. ("Happy staff – happy residents!", commented a member of staff from another home.)

The design of the home was based on the brief produced for the home opened in 1996, with only minor amendments to take account of site topography. The original project group had included suitably experienced operations managers, plus a specialist home manager, as well as design and building specialists.

As noted earlier, experience from the dementia care home which had been in operation for over six years, suggested that the quality of life for older people with dementia would be enhanced if they lived in small groups, with a staff to resident ratio not greater than 1:4. Further research and financial viability studies into groups of 8, 10 and 12 residents indicated that, for economic reasons, it was necessary to specify a group size of at least 12. The size of the home – 36 in three groups of 12 – was based on the advice of operations staff and their recommended staff:resident ratio of 1:4, and the maximum size capable of being managed effectively by one manager. (This organisation is contemplating an increase in the group size to 15 in future homes for economic reasons.)

From the first tentative discussions in 1991/2 with the authority, the home was finally opened in 1997.

Design and use of building

The home was procured using a conventional JCT form of contract. It took 13 months to build and was handed over in early November 1997. The first resident moved in during December and the home was fully occupied by September 1998. The prolongation of the process was due, in part, to the reluctance of the local social services department to refer prospective residents to the home.

The home design (Home B Plan) was based on a cruciform plan built mainly on one floor, with staff facilities, the plant room and a workshop located on a lower floor, taking advantage of the gradient of the site. The three residential wings had two groups of six resident rooms at each side of a central core containing a living room (a combined sitting and dining room with domestic scale kitchen area), two assisted bathrooms and WCs, clean linen and utility rooms and a cleaning store. The fourth wing contained mainly administration and main home service facilities. Although the kitchen areas were used by some residents, and provided therapeutic benefits, it was necessary to have a member of staff in attendance. An isolating switch linked to the cooker would have been useful.

The four wings of the cruciform met in a central foyer, set out with informal seating (Photograph 2), and used for special events for residents and visitors. The manager's office and a hairdressing room were accessed from this foyer. Staff used an electronic card system to gain access to the administration and service wing. This wing contained offices, main kitchen, laundry, two visitor bedrooms, staff meeting/training room, counselling room, with staff accommodation, storage and workshop on the lower floor. The laundry benefited from an outdoor drying terrace.

Photograph 2: A corner of the main foyer

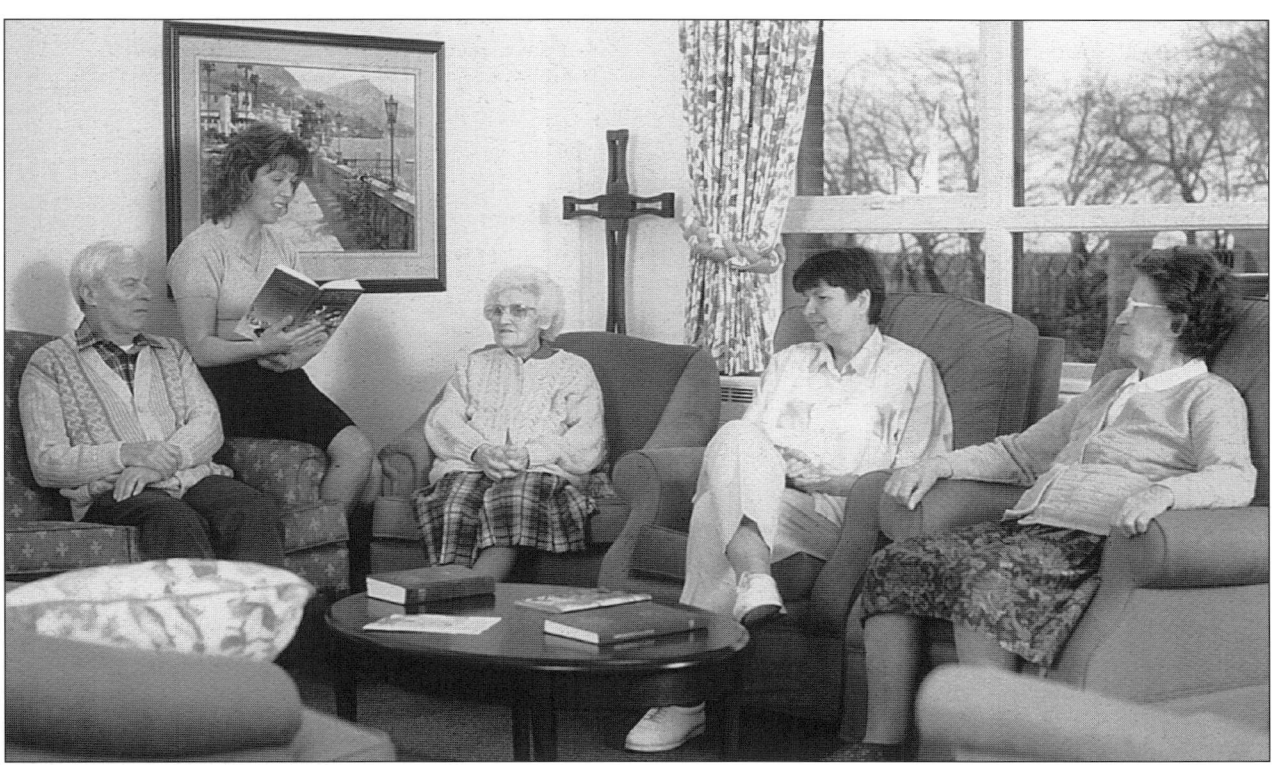

'Put yourself in my place'

Home B Plan: Ground floor

Key

aWC	Assisted toilet
B	Bedroom
b	Bathroom
Ba	Battery
be	Bench seating
Bo	Boiler
BS	Bin store
Cl	Cleaning
CSt	Cold store
D	Dining area
DB	Double guest
Dr	Drying room
DSt	Dry store
dWC	Disabled toilet
es	En suite
F	Foyer
FC	Female changing
FWC	Female staff toilets
GO	General office
GSt	General store
HD	Hairdressing
K	Main kitchen
k	Kitchen area
La	Laundry
Lin	Linen
LMR	Lift motor room
Lo	Lobby
MC	Male changing
M/C	Meeting/counselling
MO	Managers office
Mo	Mowers etc
MWC	Male staff toilets
S	Seating area
SB	Single guest/staff
Shop	Shop (used as a store)
SL	Staff lounge
T	Telephone
T/H	Training/handover
U	Utility room
VSt	vegetable store
vWC	Visitors toilet
W	Workshop
WC	Toilet

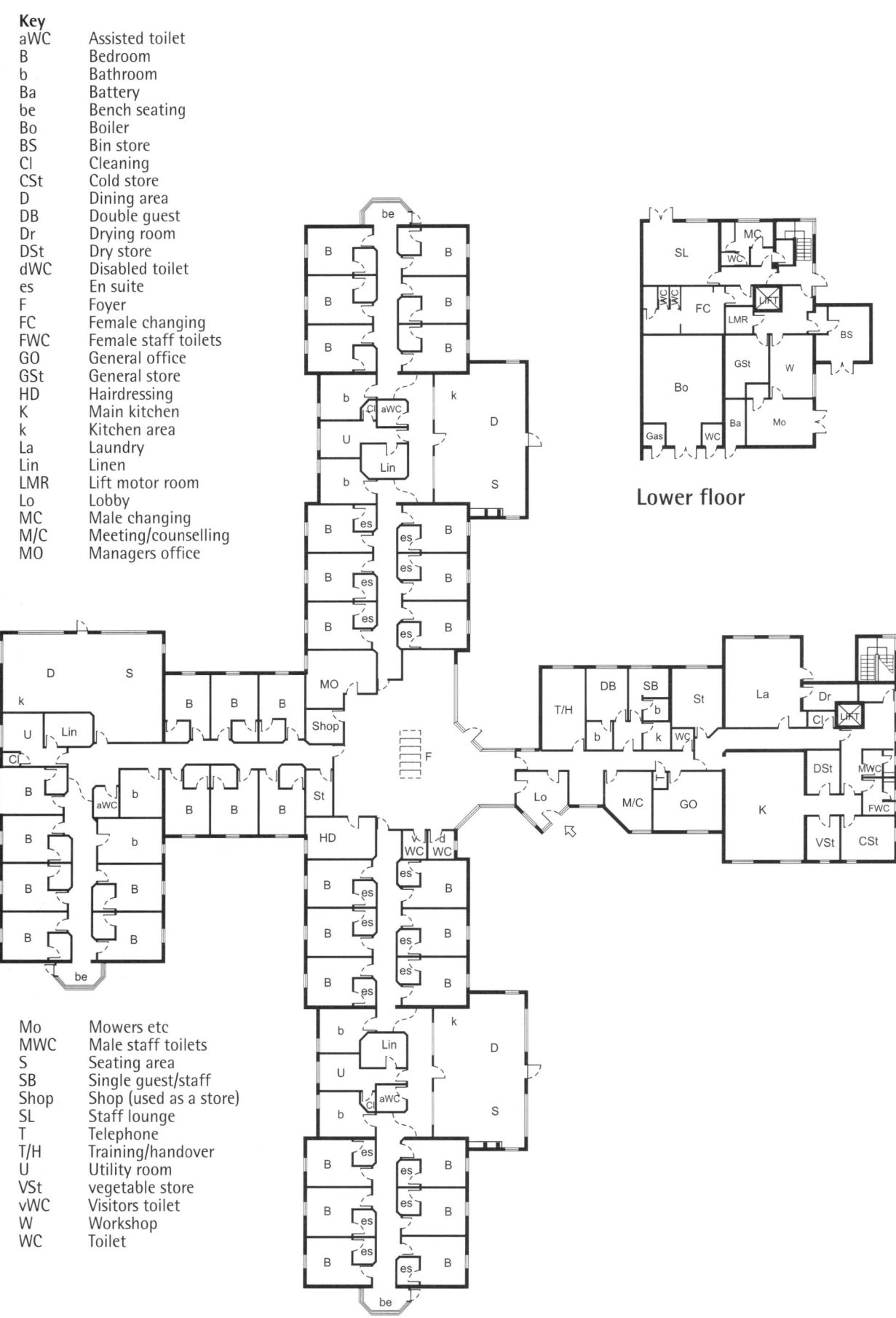

Lower floor

58

This was generous provision and reflected an attempt to create the ideal in support facilities and accommodation. The visitor bedrooms were rarely used for the purpose for which they were intended and conversion to residents' rooms was being considered.

> Consider carefully before providing dedicated guest rooms – even with a market level charge the occupancy rate may be too low.

Easy access to extensive landscaped gardens had contributed greatly to the success of the home. Access was available via doors set out of direct view at the side of seating areas at the end of each residential wing (Photograph 3), and from the living rooms. Each group had its own garden area with carefully selected planting and footpath systems, but all three gardens were linked to extend the options for exploration.

Initially, the manager considered that a combined sitting and dining room arrangement would not be suitable for the client group, but was now convinced that it worked well as it allowed residents the opportunity to move easily between the two areas and use dining tables for various activities (Photograph 4). This meant that it was possible for residents who might not initially be interested in taking part in activities to be

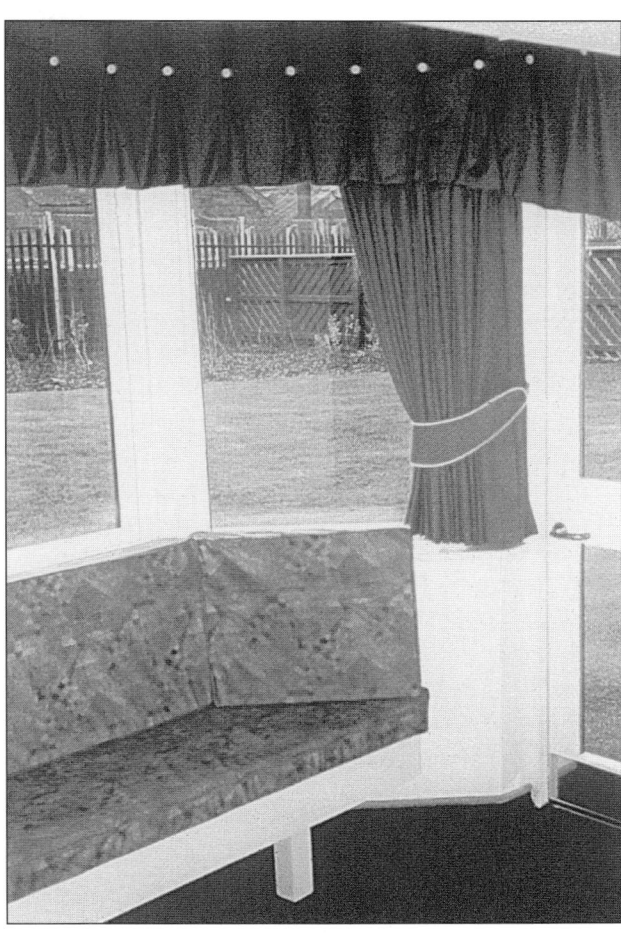

Photograph 3: Useful semi-private seating at corridor end, with fire door giving easy access to garden

Photograph 4: Dining area of a group living room – note the matching seat covering which links the dining and sitting areas

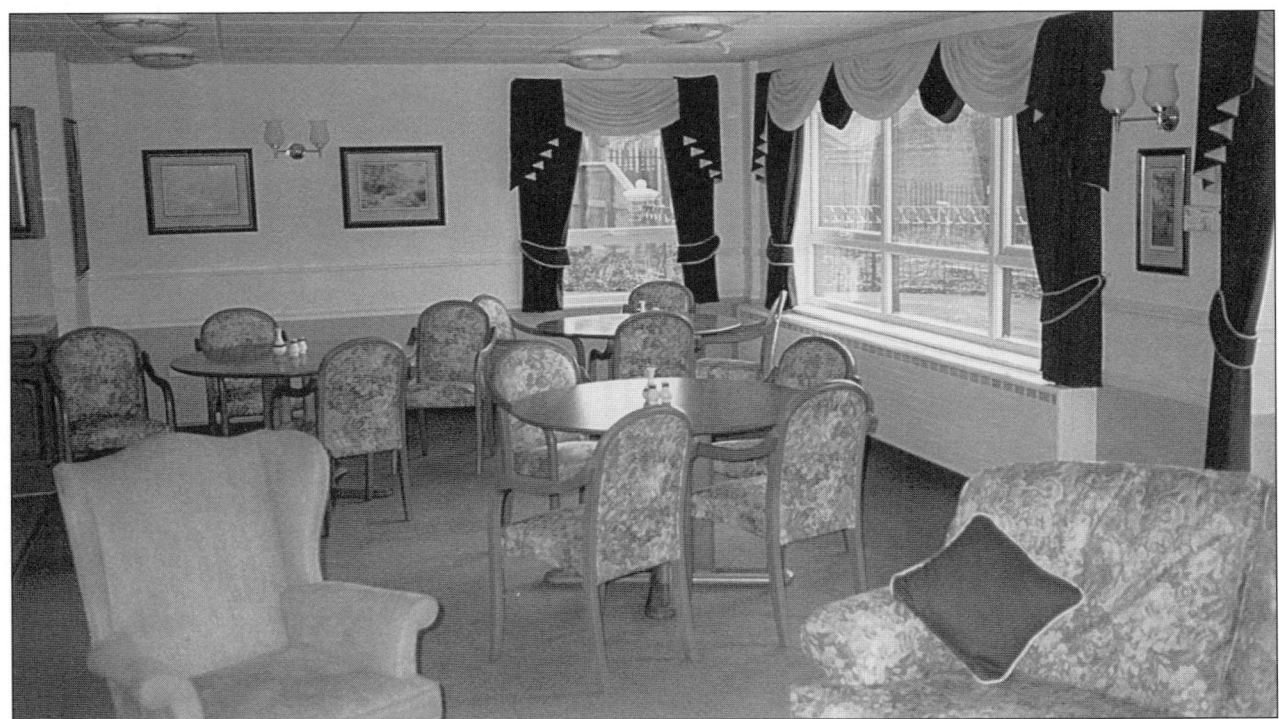

'Put yourself in my place'

attracted to the area and activity. In the same way, some residents were drawn to the kitchen areas and became involved in washing up, helping to serve meals and sometimes baking – all within view of their fellow residents. It was also easier for residents and staff to gather at tables at main meal times.

Wandering routes were not a major consideration in the design brief, as it was considered that, with appropriate stimulation, wandering could be minimised. However, routes were available within the building, linked by attractive sitting areas at the end of the residential wings, the living room and the central foyer, and to garden footpaths via easily accessible doors.

The door from the living room to the garden (fitted with a doorbell to facilitate re-entry) opened onto a large level paved terrace complete with seating and planters. The footpath systems meandered through the garden and linked with the doors at the end of the residential wings. Attractive sitting areas, complete with planted arbours, were provided along the footpaths.

A greenhouse provided an instantly recognisable feature in the garden and soft landscaping was arranged in significant groups using familiar, colourful and scented plants. It was acknowledged, however, that some raised beds would be beneficial.

The design brief also included:

- doors to the residential wings from the main foyer, colour coded to tone with the colour schemes used in the wings
- pastel coloured doors to residents' rooms, arranged so that no door opposed another
- residents' doors fitted with conventional furniture including number and letterbox (which was not used much but was a familiar feature); a framed panel for a picture or photograph was fitted at the side of the door
- attractive fire surrounds and safe coal-effect fires provided as focal points in the living rooms (Photograph 5)
- seating in a variety of styles and heights – settees were popular but were too low
- variable lighting in the living rooms to reflect a range of activities from socialising to reading or handicraft work
- increased intensity of lighting in the corridor approaches to the living rooms
- good natural light throughout the building
- centrally controlled mechanical ventilation

Photograph 5: Sitting area of a group living room with a variety of seating

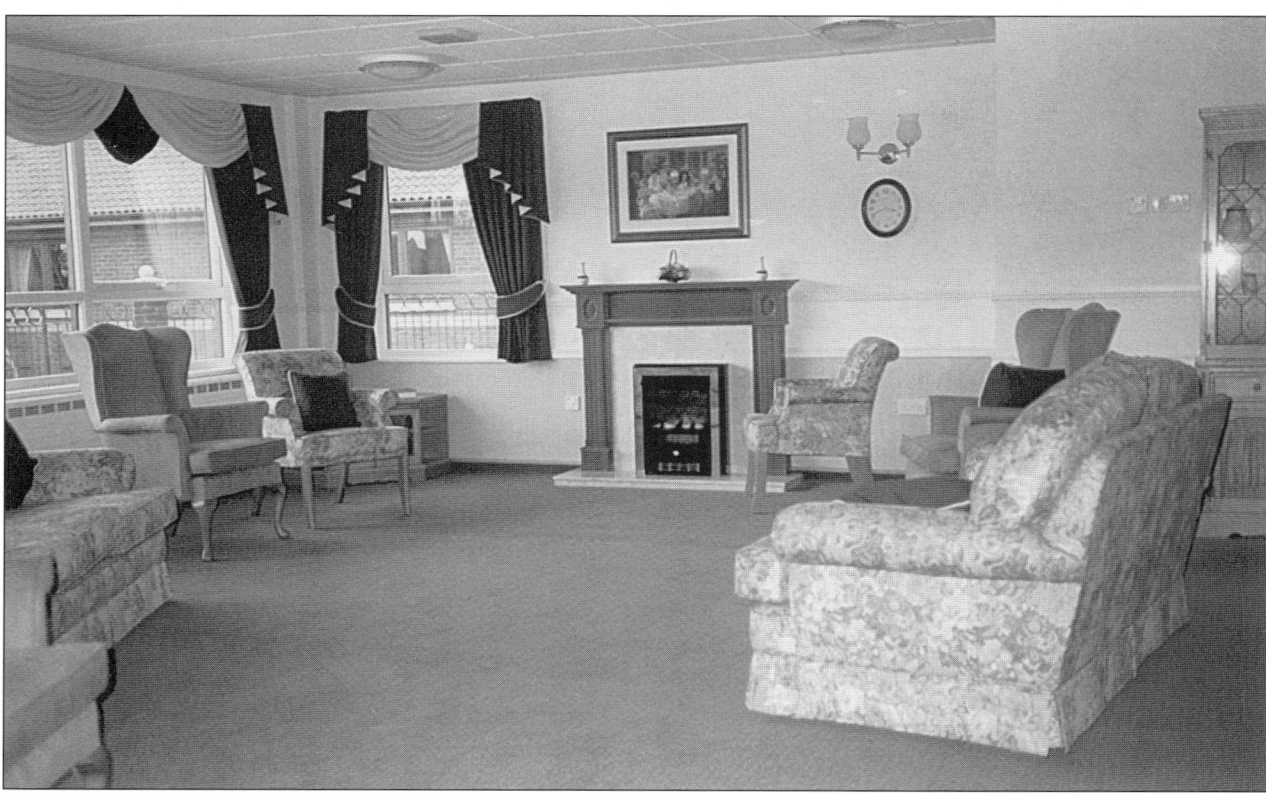

- WCs in the en suites in view from two bed positions (Photograph 6)
- secondary low intensity 'night lighting' in en suites to assist continence control.

"Anyone considering developing a care home should look at this home."

Views about Home B

Relatives

"This home provides a secure, safe environment – space."

"This home provides a stimulating environment with plenty of activities – reading etc."

Managers and care staff

"Freedom to go into the gardens is part of the success story. First floor [rooms] could be a problem with risks of using the lift. It also restricts residents' choice through staff not having time to take first floor residents out."

"Some residents dress up to go to the foyer."

"En suites are too small for hoists if needed when someone is lying on the floor."

"The bathroom without a window is not used by residents."

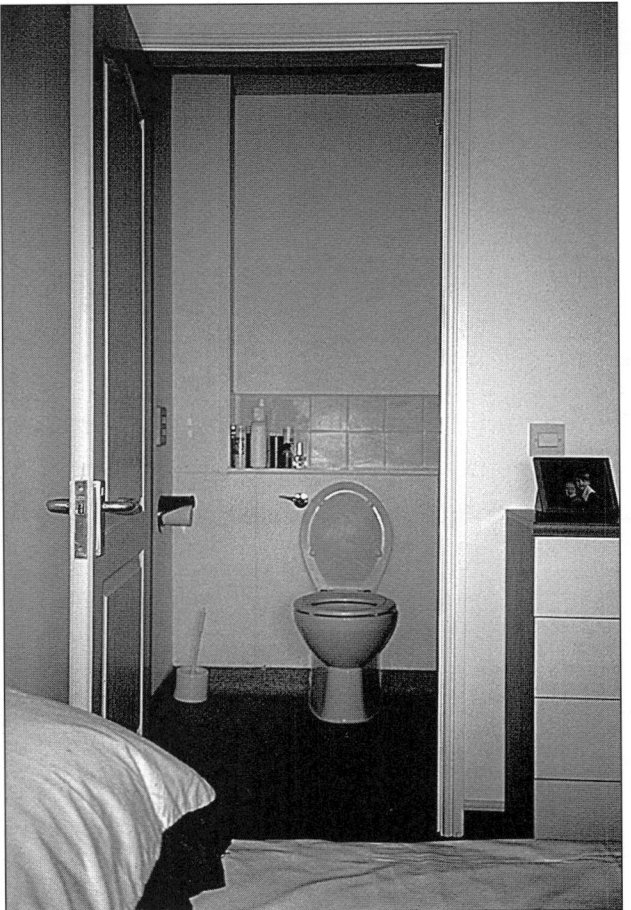

Photograph 6: WC in view from the bed with 180° door hinges and secondary low intensity lighting in en suite

Box 6.2: Design features – Home B

Enhancing features
- central foyer where all residents could gather
- single-storey building with easy access to well landscaped gardens
- living room incorporating kitchen area
- entrance arrangement enabling staff to enter and leave the home out of view of residents, thus avoiding possible distress if resident observed keyworkers leaving
- seating at ends of residential wing corridors
- interesting landscaped garden with arbours, seats and circular paths linked with clearly identified doors.

Limiting features
- too many ancillary rooms in administration wing
- lack of a dedicated quiet room
- staff facilities too far from main operational zones.

Home C

This provider, a 'not-for-profit' company, was created in 1991 when it assumed responsibility for managing over 30 residential homes from a county council. Since then, 13 homes had been re-built and most of the remainder refurbished.

An old care home in need of replacement already existed on the site on which this new 60-place residential home was eventually to be built. Thus, the demand for care was already established, supported by demographic surveys. In addition, day care facilities (all places purchased by the county council) were provided in the new home. The new building was owned by the county council and leased by the company.

Forty-four residents transferred to temporary accommodation for 14 months prior to rebuilding and 40 moved into the new home in one day in June 1996. It took a further six months to fill the remaining 20 places.

Families as well as staff were involved when residents moved into the new home. Although en suites were provided, commodes were re-introduced in the new home as it was considered that many residents would be unable to use the en suite facilities unassisted.

Design and use of building

The home was located in a suburban housing area, adjacent to a school, with a district shopping parade a short walk away. The site therefore met several basic criteria.

The company entered into a design and build contract for the home, which was completed in 12 months, within budget. The design of the new home, on two floors with two residential wings on each floor (Home C Plan), was based on previous designs and practical experience. It had an interesting symmetrical pincer-like footprint, with separate dining and sitting rooms located centrally in the angled residential wings. A small kitchen was adjacent to the dining room.

The company had developed a group-living model based on a group size of 15 and an overall home size of 60 places. The overall size was dictated by commercial necessity and the belief that this model and these sizes allowed it to meet different care needs under the same roof, but in separate groups. The overall size was the maximum allowed by the registration authority and was more cost-effective than a smaller home.

A day care unit could be linked with the entrance foyer and a sun lounge to provide an occasional meeting area for most of the residents – an enterprising means of duplicating the use of space without creating additional under-used areas.

People with dementia were located in one group of 15 on the first floor, although in the previous home completed by the company, those with dementia were located on the ground floor. The design approach, fitting out and equipment were the same for ground and first floors. No special features had been introduced in the dementia care wing. Initially it was intended that seven rooms with a dedicated dining room would be grouped together for respite care. This policy was subsequently abandoned – the segregation created administrative problems – and respite visitors were located throughout the home. It was said that "they are a breath of fresh air for the long-term residents".

> Consider carefully the provision, location, cost and staffing implications of respite rooms.

En suites were generally paired, leaving a clear floor area in the rooms, unencumbered by unproductive entrance space.

Although wandering routes were described as being freely available along corridors and stairways, at least one corridor leg in each wing was long, lacking in interest and ergonomically unsatisfactory.

A small carer station, complete with lockable medication store, was located centrally in each group unit. A dedicated hairdressing room on the first floor, situated conveniently near the lift, was much appreciated by residents and staff.

A guestroom was little used. Few homes now provide this facility, the general view being that this is a luxury that few can now afford. Generous space for staff had been provided, including a separate smoking lounge. Shared WC and shower facilities appeared to present no problems.

Home C Plan: Ground floor

Key
ab	Assisted bathroom
as	Assisted shower
aWC	Assisted toilet
B	Bedroom
Cl	Cleaning
CS	Carer station
D	Dining room
DC	Daycare
DSt	Dry store
dWC	Disabled toilet
es	En suite
F	Foyer
GO	General office
K	Main kitchen
k	Kitchenette
L	Lounge
La/I/S	Laundry/iron/sort
La/W/D	laundry/wash/dry
Lo	Lobby
MO	Managers office
R	Reception
Sl	Sluice
St	Store
Sun L	Sun lounge
SWC	Staff toilet
VSt	Vegetable store
vWC	Visitor toilet
WU	Wash up

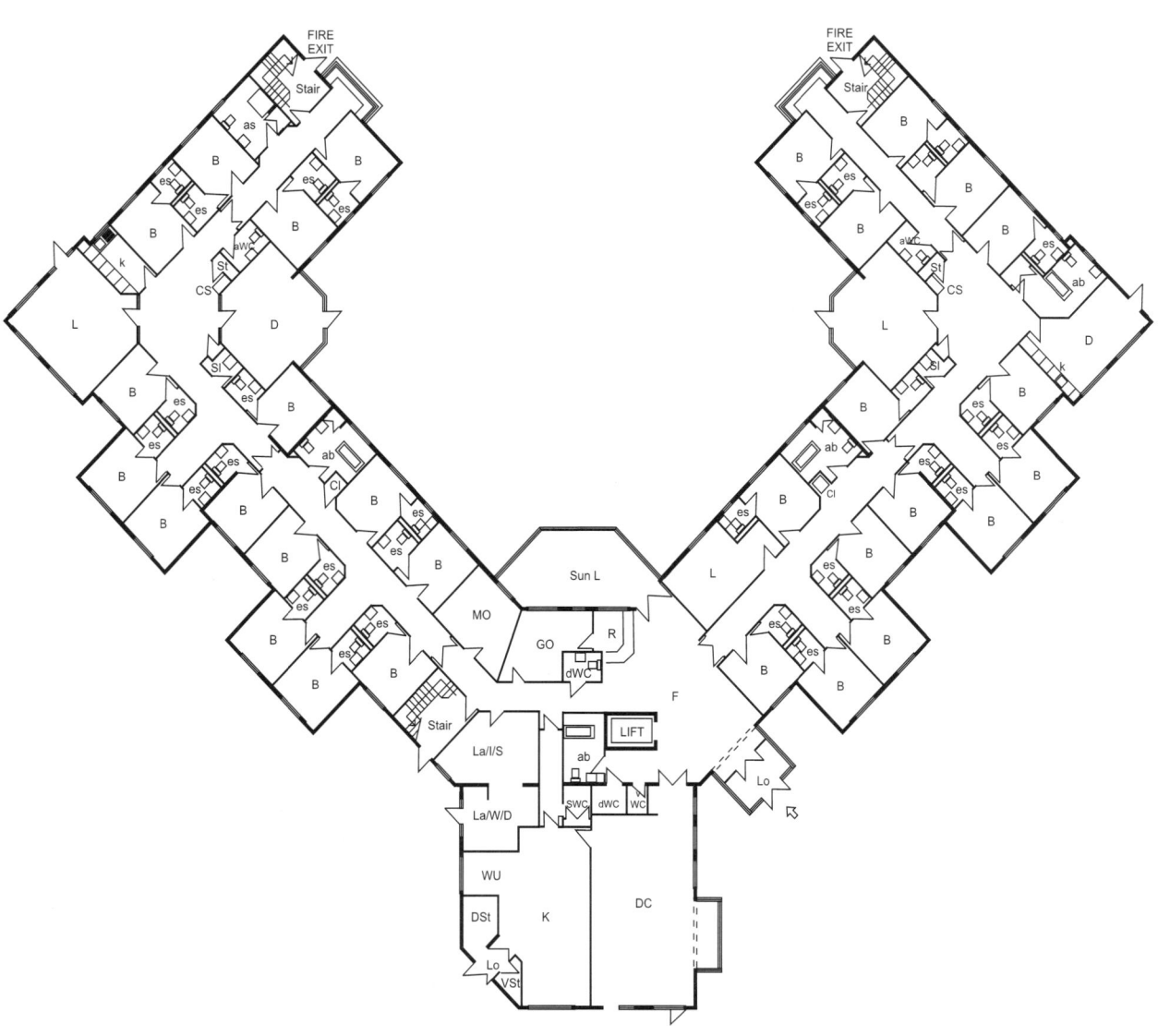

Residents had previously been in an older residential home and it appeared that few owned furniture. As a consequence the company provided resident room furniture, which, although attractive, was inevitably uniform.

Views about Home C

Residents

"I have a problem when attempting to manoeuvre my wheelchair in the en suite."

"The lack of safety features at the head of the stairs is not a problem as most residents cannot and do not attempt to use the stairs."

"The garden is an important and enjoyable feature – even if you cannot get out."

Staff

"It is useful to have a central area where all residents can meet for special occasions."

"There is a positive effect from 'mixing' residents with dementia and others."

"Outdoor drying space is available, but not used."

"We could do with air conditioning or an extraction system in corridors."

"The medication unit should be located centrally on each wing."

Relatives

"… the importance of the home being on or near a bus route."

"Attractive, interesting gardens are very important."

"Make sure that the home is built for the job – not converted – and has plenty of fresh air and light."

"Residents' rooms are not large enough to use as a sitting room [to entertain visitors in their 'own' home]." (Photograph 7)

Photograph 7: Crowding increases risk factor – allow adequate space for a walking aid and a visitor chair

Photograph 8: Wide corridor leading to bench seating and outlook over garden – but note protruding radiators and fire extinguisher

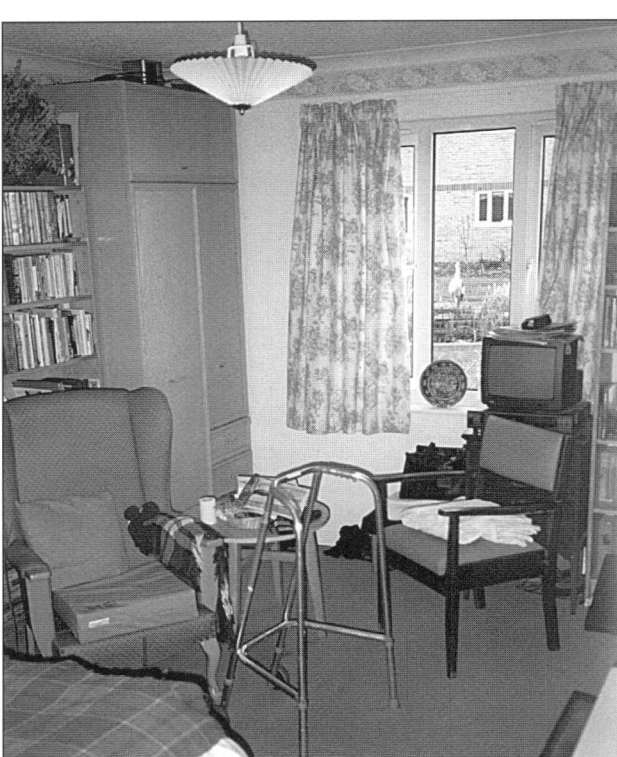
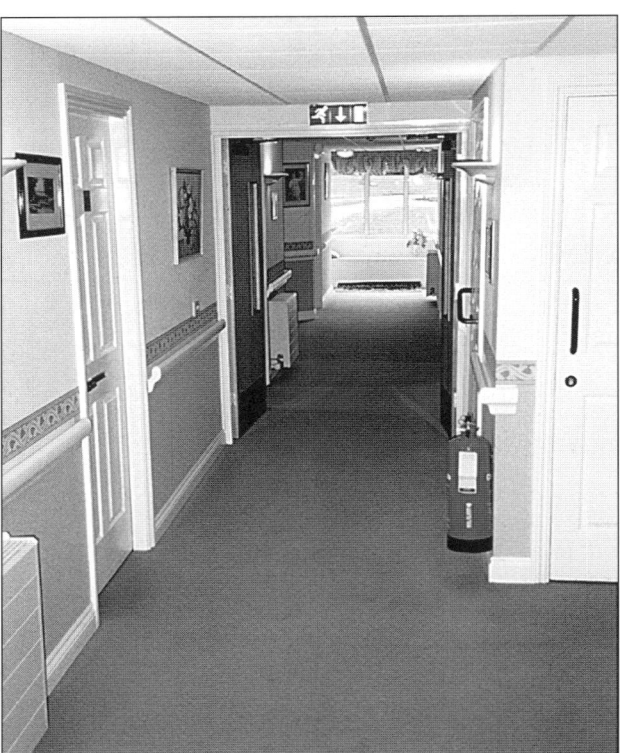

Photograph 9: Ensure adequate space available for heated trolleys

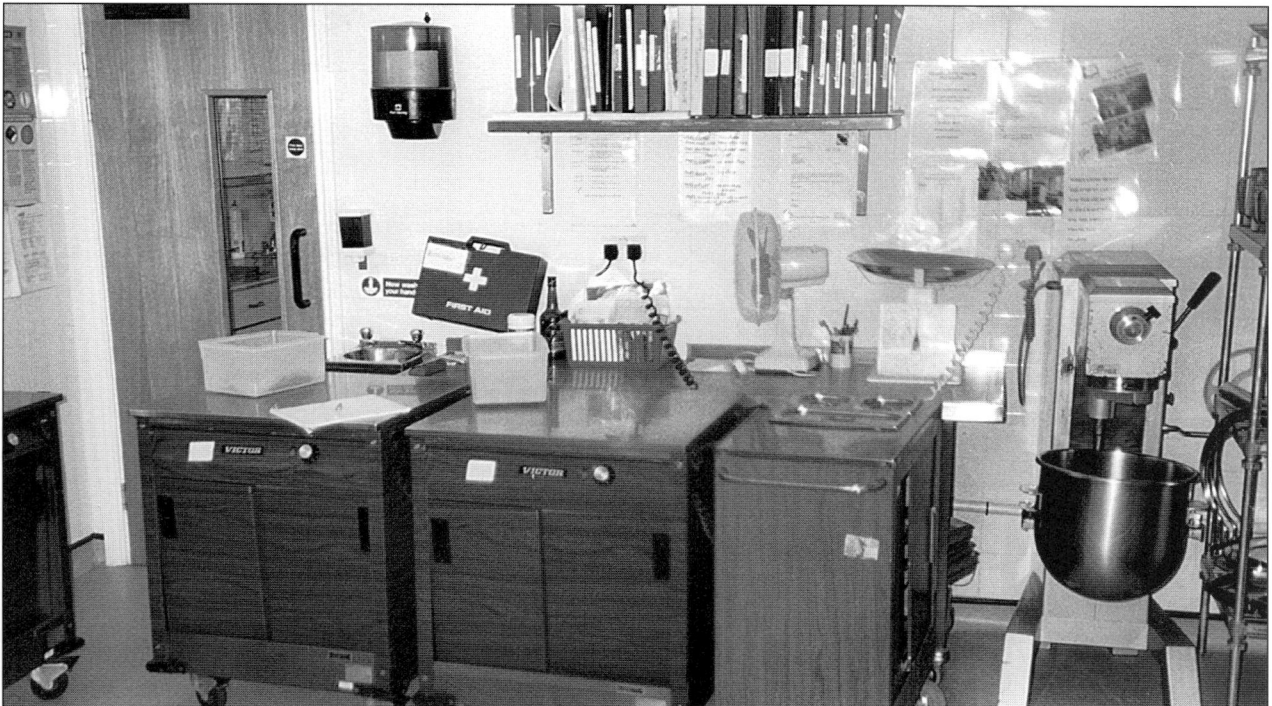

Box 6.3: Design features – Home C

Enhancing features
- room floor areas unencumbered with entrance halls or corridors and, notwithstanding the relative's comment, generally provided a clear floor space of just over 12m²
- most residents' rooms paired and separated by en suite modules, one of which was 0.6m² larger for wheelchairs and hoists
- dining room which doubled as an activity room under the guidance of a motivated activity assistant
- two large smoking lounges, one for visitors and residents and the other for staff; in addition, residents could smoke in their own rooms, after risk assessment
- generous garden areas and interesting footpath routes
- location of home in suburban area
- ability to combine day centre, entrance foyer and sun lounge to create an area for social events
- assisted bathrooms with natural light and ventilation
- bay window seating at ends of residential wings (Photograph 8)
- external doors with doorbells fitted leading from the secure garden.

Limiting features
- shortage of storage space – common complaint
- no linen store on ground floor
- lack of adequate space for heated trolleys in the kitchen (Photograph 9) and no specific storage space for fresh vegetables
- inconvenient layout of sanitary ware in en suites when manoeuvring wheelchairs or hoists, particularly when two carers were needed; WC in en suite not in view from optional bed positions
- heavy doors from assisted bathrooms and WCs opened onto corridors
- under-used assisted shower rooms – only one user
- no dedicated person responsible for the management of the laundry – consequential problems in identifying ownership of clothing
- window sills in residents' rooms too high – 750mm above floor level; a height of 675mm would enable occupants to see out of the window when in bed.

Home D

The planned closure of a long-stay psychiatric hospital for older people with severe mental health problems led to the proposal to build care homes to replace four wards.

In 1988 the health authority established a post to look into moving EMI/older people out of hospitals. The appointed person led the planning group which eventually proposed the creation of four care homes, each with a capacity of 24 places, including this home. Ninety per cent of the patients transferred to the new homes. The size of the homes, prescribed by the health authority, reflected the 24-bed size of wards in the hospital.

Unusually, two housing associations were selected to take part in the project, based on the idea that care for people with dementia could be provided more successfully in a housing model than in an institutional home model. It was two years before the housing association, which owns this home, decided to proceed with the development of two of the replacement homes. A tripartite agreement was signed with social services and the health authority, a design brief was produced and, in due course, Home D and another home were built.

Initially there were problems in persuading consultants and nursing staff to sign up to the new model – away from the hospital model of care. This may also have been because the model proposed was described as a 'housing scheme'. A booklet was subsequently produced to inform and convince GPs about the purpose of the home and to describe how the medical workload would reduce. The booklet also stated:

> "The physical environment of the nursing homes with their single-room, en suite bedrooms, well equipped communal facilities and 'age friendly' landscaping were a major factor in improving the quality of life of the study group, who were previously accustomed to wards containing up to thirty patients in the two and three storey hospital built largely at the turn of the century."

Although a nursing model of care was initially strongly supported by hospital staff and it was suspected that transfer to a residential home would have been unacceptable, care was now being provided in a dual-registered home operating what was essentially a residential model of care. The home was promoted by leaflets describing, "Apartments with specially-designed extra care facilities for older people with mental health problems".

Four sites were considered before the present site was selected as being of suitable size to accommodate a mainly single-storey 24-place unit with an acceptable garden area. The site, in a residential area, was already owned by a building company, which eventually entered into a design and build contract with the association.

The health authority awarded a significant Community Care Innovation Grant towards the capital costs of the home. The home also received significant block funding from the health authority to reflect the cost of providing high quality specialist care. Notwithstanding this, the unit cost to the health authority was still much less than the cost of care in a hospital. An additional agreement between social services and the health authority resulted in the health authority paying for nursing care.

The financial manager commented:

> "It would need a 55-place home run on the same lines and income only from social services fees for the home to be financially viable."

All financial negotiations and agreements were completed before the 1990 NHS and Community Care Act came into operation.

Design and use of building

The design brief was produced by a project team, which included the architect and quantity surveyor, as well as representatives from the housing association and the health authority. It was based on a general design brief provided by the housing association and the health authority's document 'Residential accommodation for elderly severely mentally ill people'. The design and build contractor was invited to join the project team at an early stage.

The housing association brief included the following:

- main area for all residents to meet – combined entrance area, lounge and hobbies room
- individual room size of 16m² including en suite
- separate access for staff
- conservatory – to provide variety and choice of sitting areas (Photograph 10)
- variety in gardens – use local specialist companies
- importance of storage capacity
- hard finishes to be minimised
- different colour schemes for each group wing
- avoid light coloured carpets – cleaning issue
- doors from residents' rooms to gardens – considered but rejected as a security risk
- good quality fittings for long-term benefit.

In addition, the health authority specified that they 'did not want large staff accommodation'. In the event, the accommodation provided was too small. The laundry was originally omitted from the design then added at a later date within the same overall footprint – to the detriment of the kitchen.

The home (Home D Plan) was separated from the road by the car park and landscaping. It blended unobtrusively into the street scene and had no name, just a street number.

The overall size was dictated by the requirements of the health authority – 24 places – and the preferred group size of eight specified by the housing association as 'the best solution for a family size unit'. There were two group wings for eight people on the ground floor and another on the first floor. Each wing contained a combined sitting and dining room complete with small kitchen area. The main lounge linked the conservatory and hobbies room, and short corridors on the ground floor ended in pleasant sitting areas with access to the secure garden.

Furniture, including fitted wardrobes, was provided within the design and build contract. The four en suites incorporating showers were fitted with over-large, drop-down seats in the showers and fixed showerheads (which have proved to be impractical and unpopular with residents and staff).

A provisional sum of £20,000 was allowed for landscaping and several local specialist landscape companies were invited to submit designs. The chosen design produced a continuous walk through a series of attractive, small, varied gardens in a safe environment (Photographs 11a, b, c and d).

Photograph 10: Conservatory providing useful options

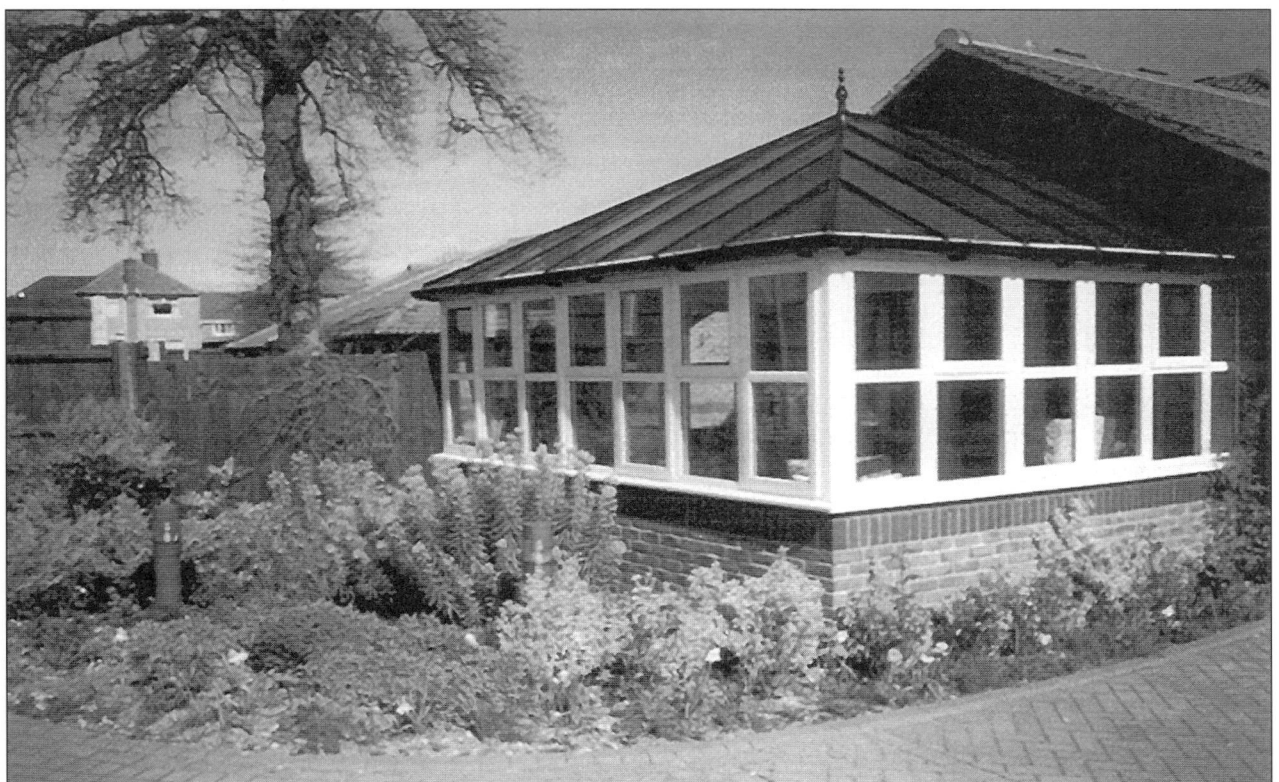

'Put yourself in my place'

Home D Plan: Ground floor

Key

aWC	Assisted toilet
B	Bedroom
ab	Assisted bathroom
C	Conservatory
Cl	Cleaning
D	Dining area
DrSt	Drug store
dWC	Disabled toilet
ES	External storeroom
es	En suite
GST	General store
H	Hobbies room
Int On	Interview/overnight
K	Main kitchen
L	Lounge
La	Laundry
Lin	Linen
Lk	Staff lockers
Lo	Lobby
MA	Meeting area
O	Office
R	Reception
Sh	Shower
S	Sitting room
Staff	Staff room
WC	Toilet
W/C	Wheelchair store
WU	Wash up

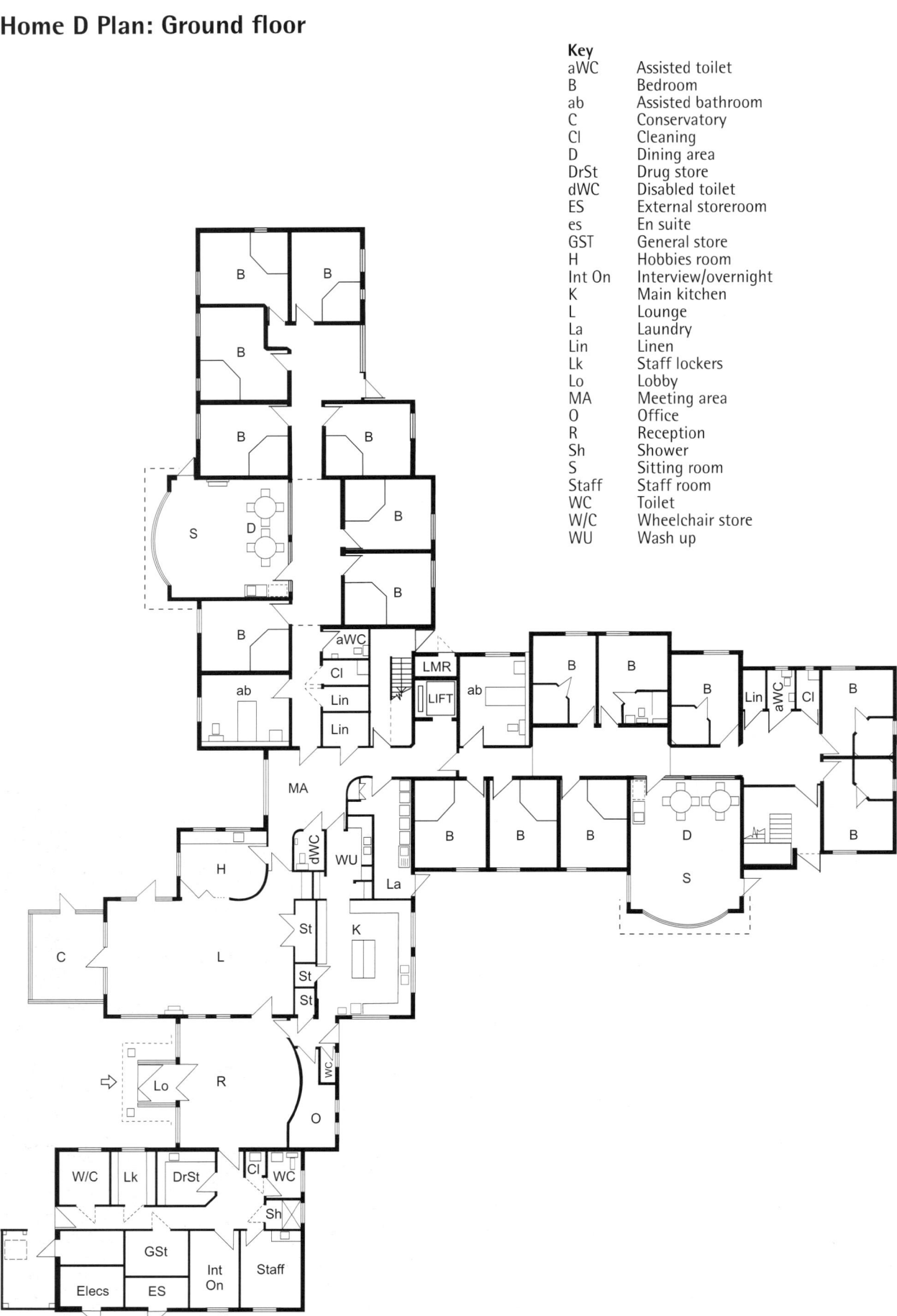

Views about Home D

Relatives

"An advice centre is needed to advise on routes to take and select the best financial report – got the illness to cope with, *don't* need the extra worry of financial burden." (From a spouse who had experienced severe difficulties)

Relatives also identified the following as particularly important features of a new home:

- security
- own en suite – preserves dignity
- purpose-built with small groups and natural light
- good use of private, semi-private, public space
- purposeful routes – no cul-de-sacs
- stimulation facilities.

Home manager

"Avoid separate dining room [splits staff and under-uses space]."

"Problem with fully-tiled bathrooms – voice timbre changes may confuse residents."

On bed-sitting rooms: "bedrooms hardly used during the day".

"Residents are attracted to activity areas – but the challenge is to create meaningful activity."

"Avoid small rooms for different activities – a single large room is better."

Staff

Staff have expressed the following views:

- attraction of community setting for home
- prefer group of eight to larger group (but no real experience of larger groups)
- importance of group-living system for easier bonding
- wardrobes in residents' rooms too small
- showers in en suites, with wheeled chair as necessary, would be beneficial
- WC in en suite too close to wall
- under-floor heating unsuitable for older people
- no air change system
- staff accommodation too limited and no training area.

Photographs 11a-d: Features from the same garden offering areas of variety and interest

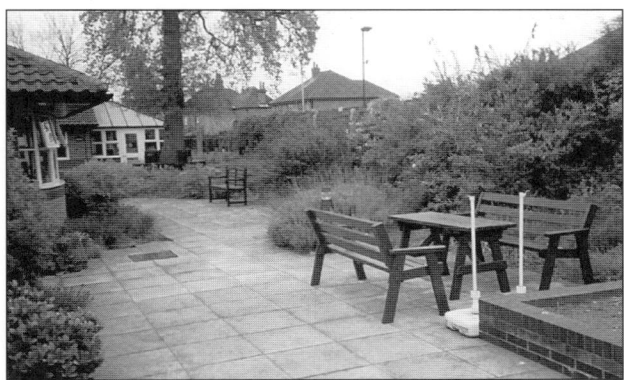
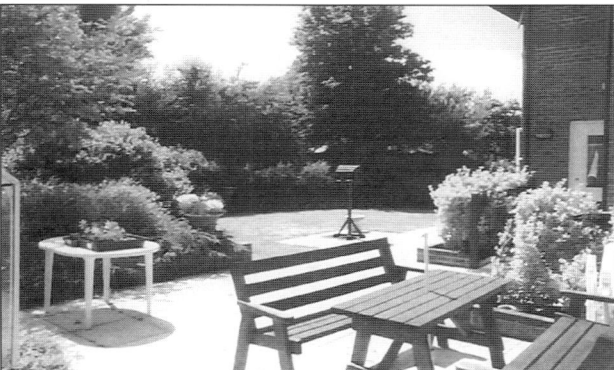
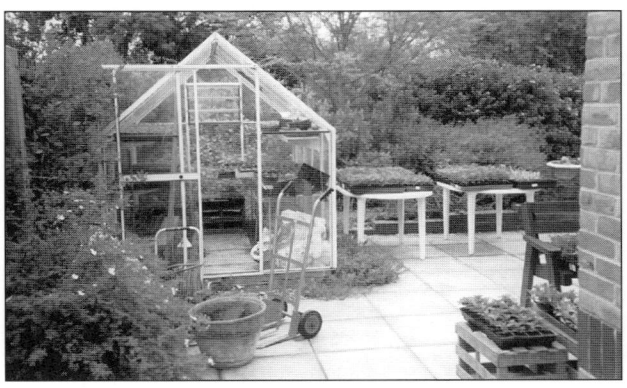
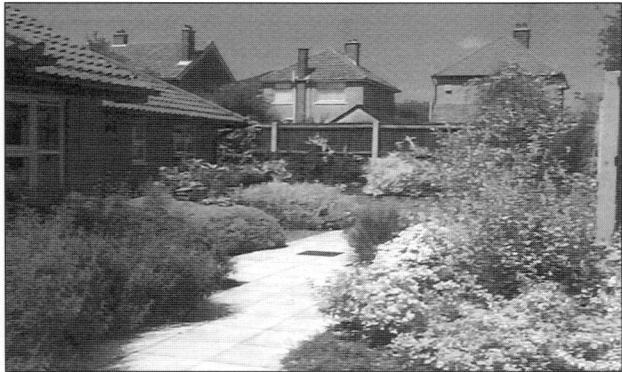

County council

"I would have liked resident rooms bigger."

"Clues for residents important."

"Perhaps this scheme is too big?"

"Personal space is important."

"We have tried to give people as domestic a setting as possible."

"The building's design restricts wandering around corridors and front entrance."

"We favour a group size of eight and believe that anything above ten will affect staff resident relationships."

"The residents' quality of life improved [from hospital to home] even though progressive dementia continued."

"Increased standards bring increased costs."

"There is no reason why people with dementia should not have same environmental quality as anyone else."

Photograph 12: Useful corridor seating but perhaps problems with fire regulations and access to handrail

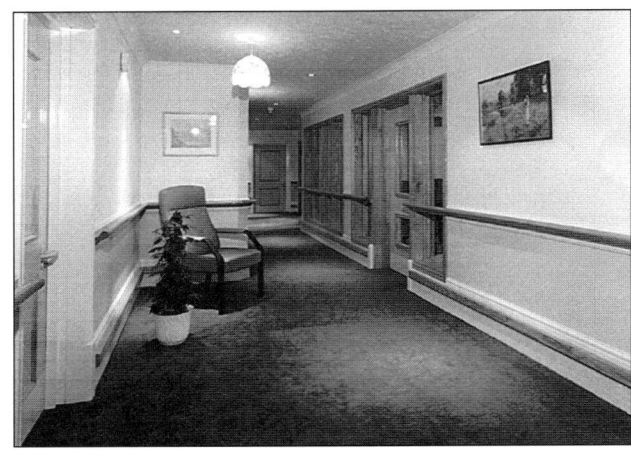

Box 6.4: Design features – Home D

Enhancing features
- small groups
- the conservatory, which was well used and provided an additional quiet room
- the hobbies room – used five days a week with the incorporated hairdressing facility being used twice a week
- secure garden area
- varied colour schemes
- separate access for staff, away from view of residents, who might be distressed to see keyworker leaving
- dual-purpose interview room, occasionally used by relatives for overnight stays
- payphone for staff and visitors, with cordless 'phones on each wing used by residents
- occasional furniture located in recesses enhanced the corridors (Photograph 12)
- a generous budget allowance was allocated for garden maintenance – and was effectively used.

Limiting features
- service delivery to kitchen by hand – kitchen access at rear of building
- restricted access to building after a resident fell on the stairs, at which point high level baffle handles were temporarily fitted to doors
- free-standing desk in entrance foyer – isolated and little used
- shortage of general storage space
- storage of continence pads, staff records and other items in wheelchair store
- storage of old medical records in drug store
- kitchen too small – no planned space for trolleys
- laundry not big enough – maybe an issue of shape as well as size
- administration space and staff rest rooms small
- wardrobes small
- location of assisted bathrooms – would have been better located in the middle of the wing
- resident doors all the same finish and colour; apparently this did not present problems, although it was acknowledged that some form of personal feature – photograph or picture – might be helpful
- heating system comprising a combination of floor and ceiling heating methods which, despite meeting performance specification, was unpopular with staff and residents who had a perception of 'hot floors'; perhaps their dislike stemmed from the lack of visible heating units such as radiators
- call system difficult for people with dementia to recognise, requiring staff to be more vigilant
- window sills too high; a height of 675mm above floor level would enable occupants to see out of window when in bed.

Home E

This organisation was established in 1992 as an Industrial and Provident association with charitable status and, after protracted negotiations with the local authority, took over 24 homes with 1,000 residents. Negotiations were complicated because the local authority changed the funding arrangements at a late stage and, in addition, 12 months later four unitary authorities replaced the original local authority, with different ideas on revenue funding. In preparing its policy for refurbishing the homes, the provider set a threshold figure so that, if refurbishment were to cost more than £12,000 per place, the home would have to be replaced.

A project group prepared a design brief which determined the size of the home. It had to accommodate 'about 80' residents from homes due for closure, and it had to be a single-storey building. Before the search for a site commenced in earnest, an operational model for the home, together with budget estimates, was produced, and this dictated the size of the site.

The search for a suitable site large enough to accommodate the proposed home centred on the catchment for existing homes. Eventually a local authority-owned site, located in an area identified for a new community, was found. It took three years to purchase this site – much longer than anticipated. Once building was completed, the move from homes that were to be closed to the new home took three weeks.

Design and use of building

The experience of the designers originally appointed proved to be inadequate and they were replaced by architects with specialist knowledge in designing care homes.

Based on the specification produced by the project group and a staff:resident ratio dictated by the operational management of 1:8, a group size of 24 was determined. It also related neatly to regulatory requirements for assisted bathrooms of 1:8 residents and WCs at 1:4.

The resultant design (Home E Plan) comprised three linked single-storey, quadrangle-style bungalows. Each provided 24 resident places and was capable of being operated independently, although sharing common facilities such as kitchen and laundry. Two bungalows each accommodated 24 residents with dementia.

In addition to the foregoing, operational managers had clear views based on the shortcomings of old buildings and, among other features, identified the need for a suitable wandering route. This was achieved by a continuous walkway within each bungalow. The three bungalows were also connected by an attractive 'street' which formed the primary circulation route for the home around the central courtyard. It contained common facilities such as a hairdresser, meeting room, manager's office and a shop. It also provided attractive seating and display alcoves for memorabilia (Photograph 13).

Photograph 13: 'The street' with seating which overlooks the central courtyard ...

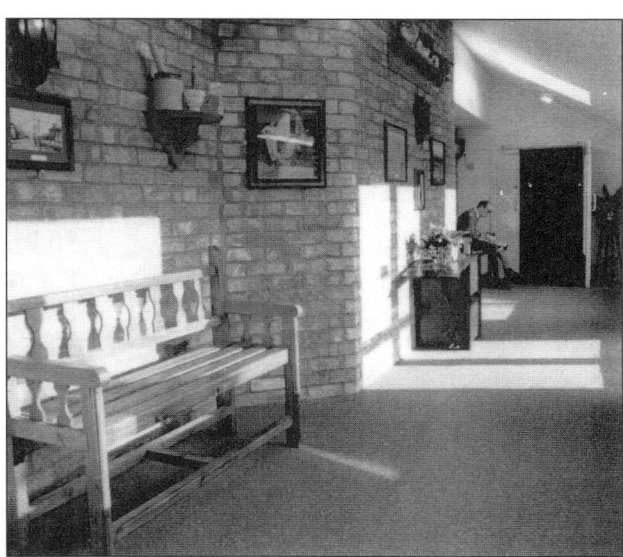

'Put yourself in my place'

Home E Plan: Ground floor

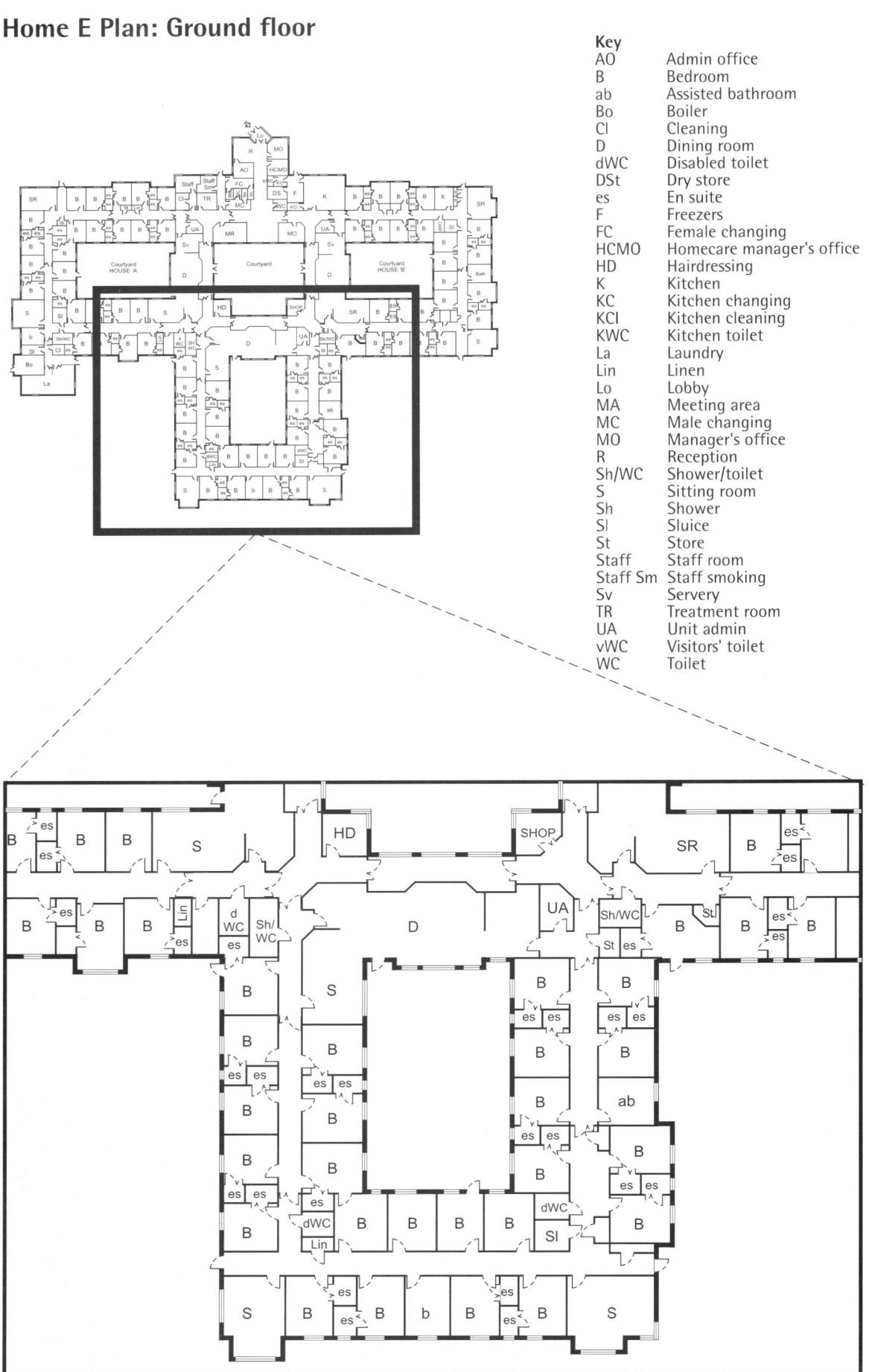

Key
AO	Admin office
B	Bedroom
ab	Assisted bathroom
Bo	Boiler
Cl	Cleaning
D	Dining room
dWC	Disabled toilet
DSt	Dry store
es	En suite
F	Freezers
FC	Female changing
HCMO	Homecare manager's office
HD	Hairdressing
K	Kitchen
KC	Kitchen changing
KCl	Kitchen cleaning
KWC	Kitchen toilet
La	Laundry
Lin	Linen
Lo	Lobby
MA	Meeting area
MC	Male changing
MO	Manager's office
R	Reception
Sh/WC	Shower/toilet
S	Sitting room
Sh	Shower
Sl	Sluice
St	Store
Staff	Staff room
Staff Sm	Staff smoking
Sv	Servery
TR	Treatment room
UA	Unit admin
vWC	Visitors' toilet
WC	Toilet

Each bungalow was accessed from the 'street' and each dining room (Photograph 14) overlooked it and the central courtyard. The main sitting room for each bungalow overlooked a secondary courtyard, and there were two other sitting rooms situated at the extreme corners of the bungalows. All resident rooms were designed for single occupation but each bungalow contained a pair of rooms with an interconnecting door for couples. Corridors were wide enough to accommodate the usual traffic involving wheelchairs, zimmer frames and those who needed a carer's assistance.

Two assisted bathrooms and an assisted shower room served each bungalow of 24 residents producing a ratio of 1:8 residents. Although the shower room was not used much, effectively making the ratio 1:12, this apparently did not cause difficulties.

Photograph 14: ... and the linked dining room – note the good design of chairs with arms which extend over the front legs providing strength at the rising leverage point

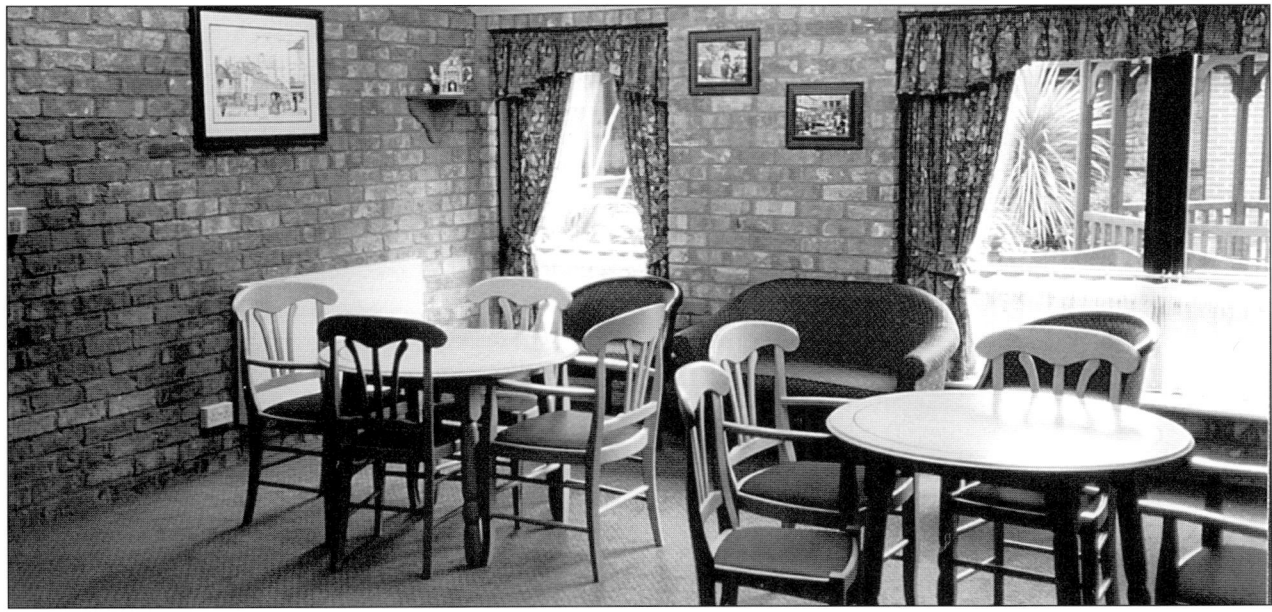

Photograph 15: Special features enhance the enclosed courtyard

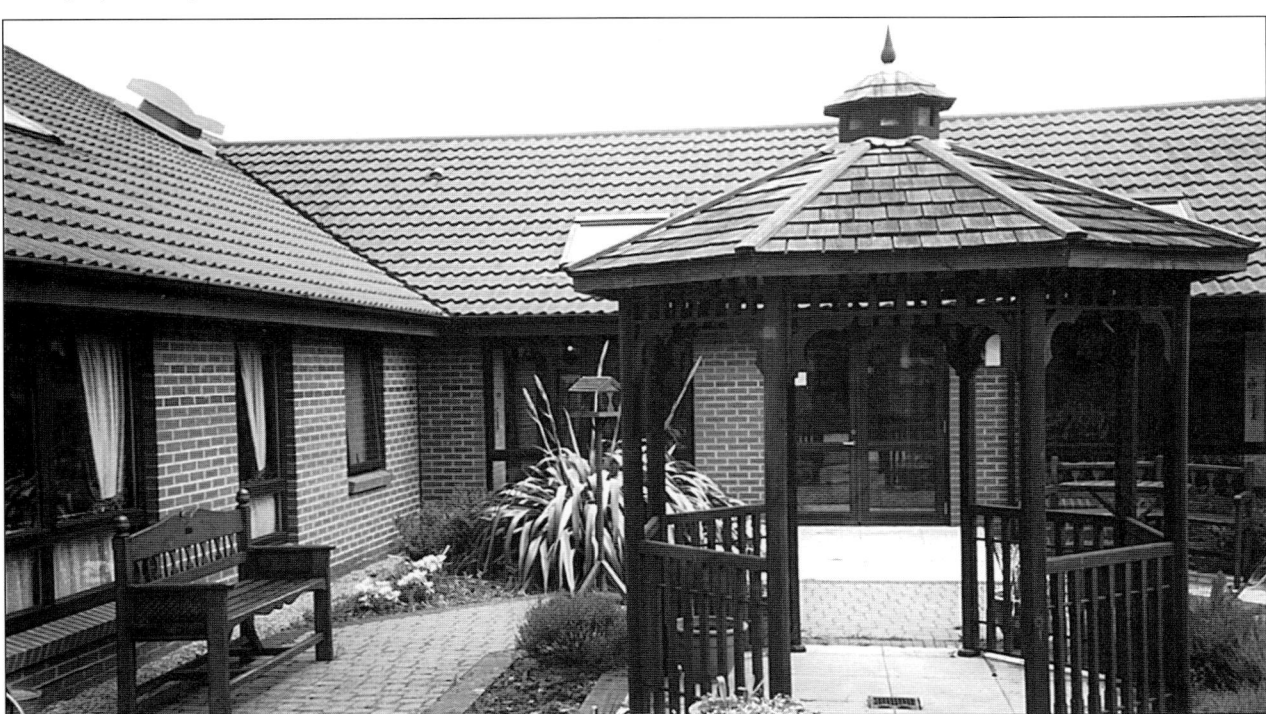

Views about Home E

Staff

"The design of the building involves staff in a lot of walking to carry out their duties."

"The servery needs ventilation."

"The lack of mechanical ventilation in bathrooms results in steaming up and overheating; if the window is opened, there is a draught."

"There is a lack of space for all residents to meet."

Box 6.5: Design features – Home E

Enhancing features
- 'street' concept with shop fronts and reminiscence areas
- courtyards – easily visible to residents, well landscaped and attractive with seating and, in the central courtyard, a pagoda (Photograph 15)
- attractive exposed facing bricks in the 'street' created a warm effect enhanced by the addition of memorabilia and pictures
- wandering routes and, in particular, the route following the 'street' around the central courtyard
- alarmed doors giving access to the external garden area; although originally there was no restriction, experience had indicated that monitoring was essential
- central kitchen – access for deliveries was good and distribution of hot meals to the serveries operated satisfactorily
- two staff rest rooms were provided – one for smokers
- resident room furniture was provided but residents could bring their own if they wished
- involvement of relatives in the choice of furniture, fittings and soft furnishings, which was possible because residents were being transferred from other homes.

Limiting features
- resident room sizes limiting for wheelchair users – despite being based on the registration standard of 10m² plus 'a bit' – 10.8m², excluding en suites where provided
- only one identified bed position – most residents had located their beds away from the normal range of services
- three sitting rooms for 24 residents, resulting in staff constantly on the move to cover all residents; to overcome this, residents were often gathered in only one or two rooms but this limited space for visitors
- shortage of storage space – in common with other homes visited, for example, for old personal records and garden furniture
- shortage of parking space for walking aids in the dining rooms – resulting in staff spending time moving or collecting aids
- no meeting space for *all* residents to gather
- splendid shop unit complete with signboard on the 'street' – not used by residents
- long and relatively uninteresting corridor route around each bungalow; also as it was difficult to provide suitable cueing devices it could be confusing to residents
- fire extinguishers projecting into corridor could be hazardous
- restricted access to WCs in en suites for hoists or wheelchairs – despite provision of additional narrow opening door
- no special cueing on doors to residents' rooms – only a small plate with a room number and space for a name card; coloured doors now being considered, with panels for photographs or pictures
- conventional assisted baths no longer user-friendly – to be replaced eventually with more user-friendly models
- residents were not encouraged to use the serveries – possibly an opportunity lost for stimulating activity
- lack of ventilation in internal areas
- large roof overhang, making some resident rooms dark
- window sills 750mm above floor level resulted in a finished height to the glazing of 800mm; while avoiding the need for toughened glass, this meant that the sill was above eye level when a resident was in bed.

Home F

This provider was a charity founded over a thousand years ago. Now registered with The Housing Corporation, it provided housing and care home accommodation for older people.

In 1990 the charity built and opened a nursing home and also undertook an extensive study into the needs of older people in its operating area. The findings of this study, and further research and discussion with the Dementia Services Development Centre, Stirling, resulted in an excellent detailed design brief. The CADE model, with clusters of rooms around central communal areas allowing total visual access, was considered best able to meet the needs of the potential client group. However, the finished design was significantly modified from the preferred model as a consequence of site constraints and fire regulations.

The charity was determined to locate the home in an urban setting on the fringe of a city so that it would meet community-based needs and would also be more accessible for visitors. A site already partly owned by the charity was selected, within walking distance of local shopping and associated facilities.

> When choosing a site, consider the needs and potential influence of the community, as well as the proximity of shops and bus services.

Although consideration was given initially to the development of a residential home, it was eventually registered as a Mental Nursing Home. The home achieved full occupancy within two weeks and operated for a year before the incorporated day centre was opened.

A design and build contract was utilised through an associated development company, thus avoiding the need to pay VAT on professional fees.

The capital cost of the project was funded from the charity's own funds and, in addition, careful budgeting for household items such as curtains, furniture, cutlery, crockery, cleaning equipment and toilet paper, ensured that there were no surprises.

In addition, a substantial subsidy was required each week from the charity to cover the shortfall in income arising from inadequate social security fee levels. The weekly expenditure was set to rise as the shortage of suitably qualified and experienced staff increased, and imposed legislation added to costs.

Design and use of building

The brief specified the size of the home to be:

> "A minimum of 20 beds ... but with more if possible up to a maximum of 30." (26 beds were provided)

The key objective was:

> "... to create a homely rather than a clinical atmosphere, mindful in all respects of the particular needs of those suffering from dementia."

In addition it stated that:

> "Ideally, each unit [sub-groups of residents] should give residents total visual access to all that they require, and, in particular, the rooms in each unit should have immediate access to a communal area combining dining and sitting facilities for each unit."

The brief also included a requirement for a day centre to serve other needs in the community.

Initially, an architectural competition was arranged involving three local firms and a national practice. The latter was successful because of a more demonstrable understanding of the needs of the client group and the principles that lay behind the design brief.

The design (Plan – Home F) made full and effective use of the restricted site. The main curved frontage of the home adjoined a busy road in an urban location but had an attractive intimate entrance on a side road. An equally attractive landscaped and secure courtyard garden, bordered by a stream, was located at the rear and incorporated a distinctive arbour walk, terraces and low walls for pots and troughs (Photographs 16 and 17). Doors could be left open to allow residents to come and go into the garden.

Home F Plan: Ground floor

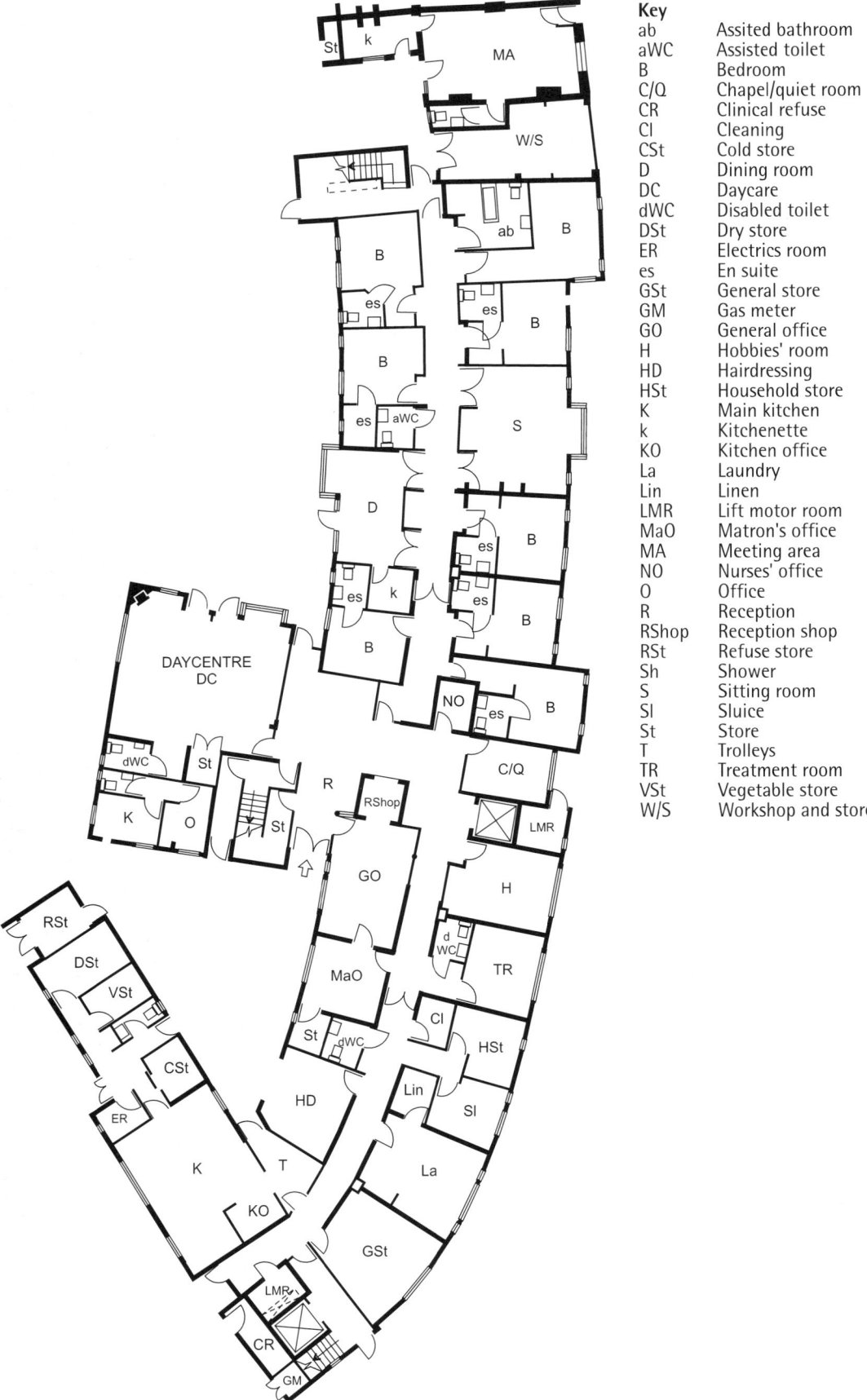

Key
ab	Assited bathroom
aWC	Assisted toilet
B	Bedroom
C/Q	Chapel/quiet room
CR	Clinical refuse
Cl	Cleaning
CSt	Cold store
D	Dining room
DC	Daycare
dWC	Disabled toilet
DSt	Dry store
ER	Electrics room
es	En suite
GSt	General store
GM	Gas meter
GO	General office
H	Hobbies' room
HD	Hairdressing
HSt	Household store
K	Main kitchen
k	Kitchenette
KO	Kitchen office
La	Laundry
Lin	Linen
LMR	Lift motor room
MaO	Matron's office
MA	Meeting area
NO	Nurses' office
O	Office
R	Reception
RShop	Reception shop
RSt	Refuse store
Sh	Shower
S	Sitting room
Sl	Sluice
St	Store
T	Trolleys
TR	Treatment room
VSt	Vegetable store
W/S	Workshop and store

'Put yourself in my place'

Photograph 16: Attractive feature providing interest and planting opportunities for a small garden ...

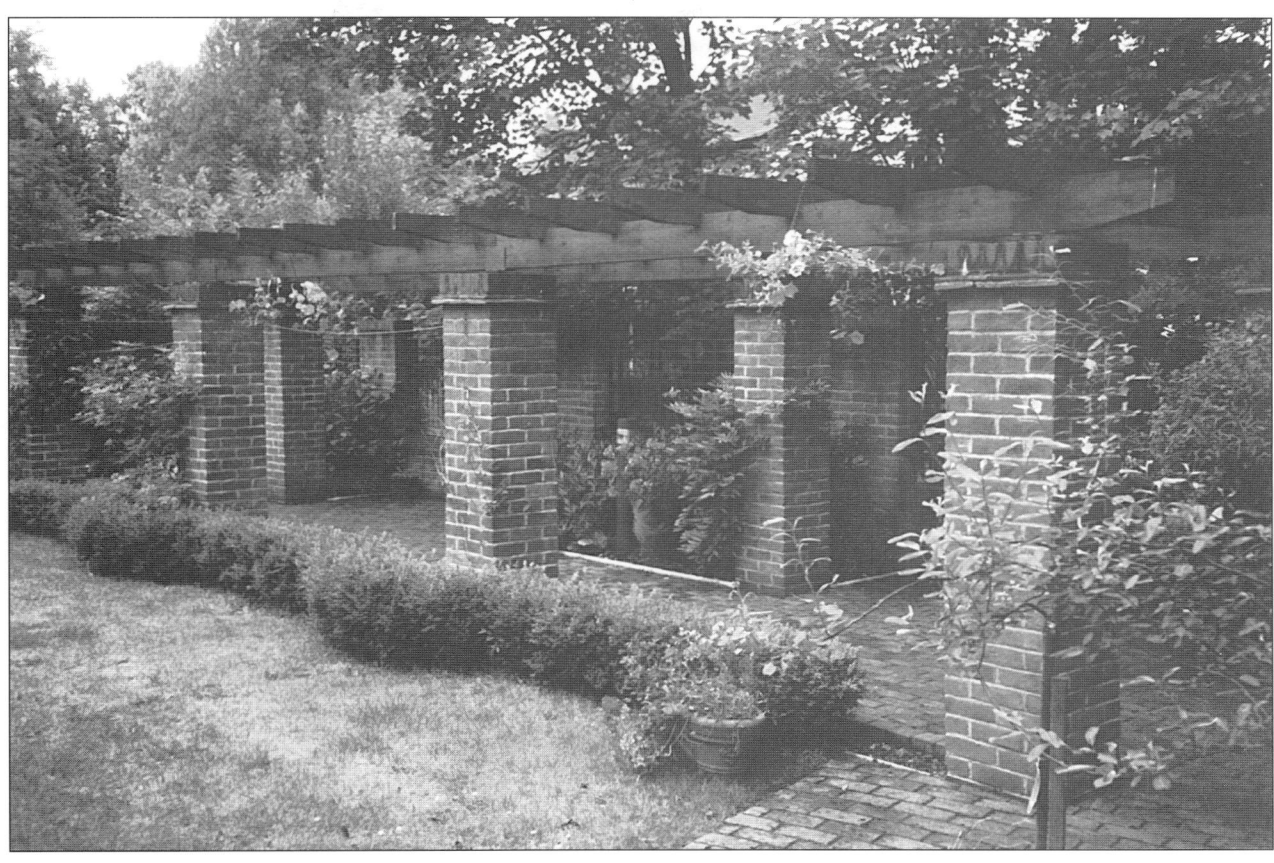

Photograph 17: ... and another small area, which was also full of interest – note the alternative to a raised garden

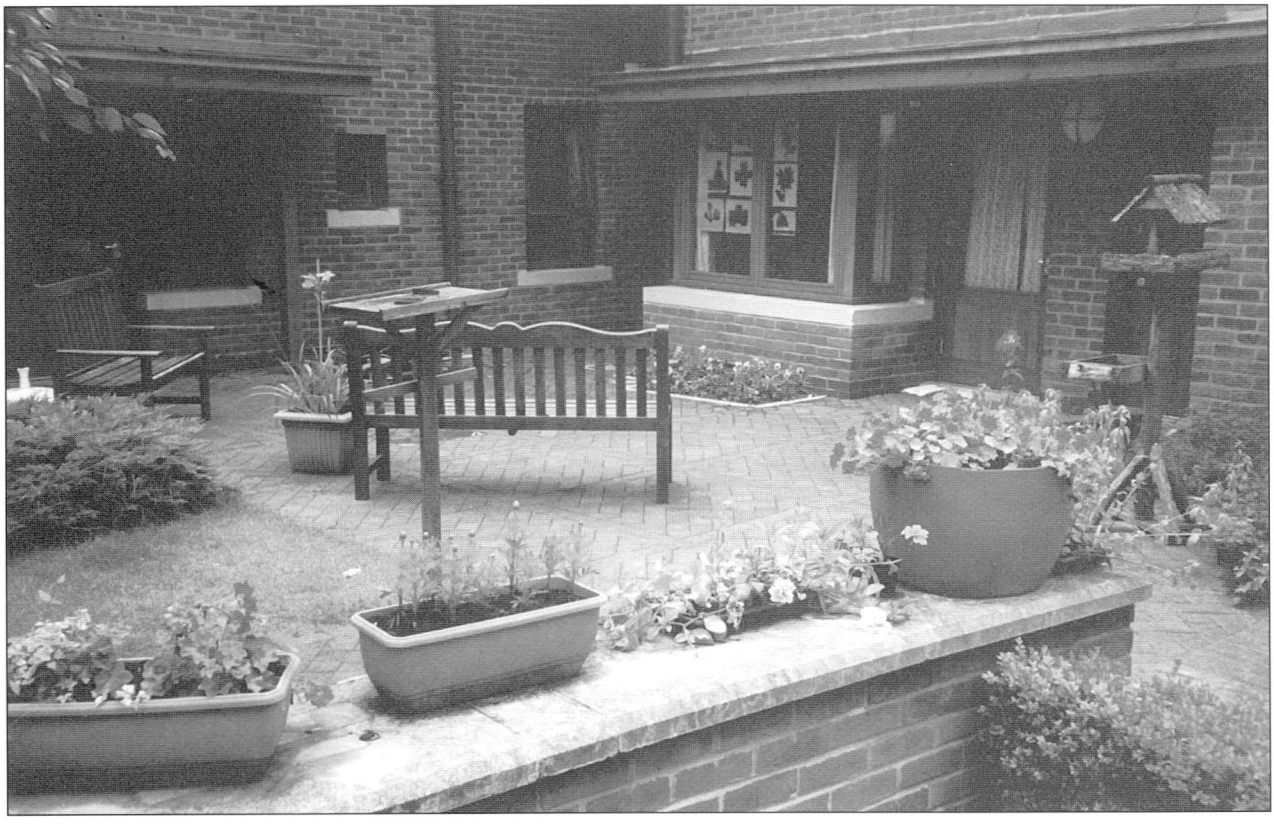

> Do not be deterred by a site which is apparently too small – a suitably experienced architect will advise on what is possible.

The home provided accommodation on two floors for 23 long-term residents and three in respite or assessment beds. The plan was in a T-form with two main groups of eight and one of seven. The brief specified a maximum group size of eight. The main groups were served by separate sitting and dining rooms. An additional bedroom for use as a guest room was provided in the roof space, which also contained the central boilers and an air-handling plant, thus freeing valuable space on the lower floors.

The respite group was provided with a small separate living/dining room and a bathroom but, as respite visitors tended to gravitate to one of the adjoining groups for meals and company, this was regarded now as part of their respite care.

In the main, there was a homely atmosphere, although hospital beds and hospital-style tables with minimal personal furniture created an austere effect. However, residents' rooms tended to be used only as bedrooms, with residents gathering in the day rooms. The location of the dining and sitting rooms centrally on opposite sides of the curved corridors shortened the effective length of corridors and improved cueing. A nurses' office was located centrally on each floor.

Intimate seating areas were strategically placed on the ground and first floors from which residents could observe routine daily movements and, in addition, a chapel (also used as a quiet room) was prominently located on the ground floor.

Planned wandering routes were deliberately excluded from the brief and residents were free to roam in the home. The corridor and residents' rooms on each floor were linked with same-coloured carpets, thus overcoming the potential problem for people with dementia created by contrasting floor colours. While this produced a bland effect to the eye, expecting distinctive, but sensitive, definition between the semi-public corridor and the private rooms, it was apparently helpful to residents.

Generous staff facilities were provided in a location which allowed them to relax away from their routine care work. The home's main service facilities were contained in a single-storey wing along a secondary street frontage, including the main kitchen, which provided all meals, and the laundry. The laundry shape and size were satisfactory, although hanging space was inadequate.

Signage in the home was minimal, while complying with statutory requirements, but large panels on residents' room doors allowed them to display familiar messages, drawings or photographs (Photograph 18). Differentiation, by means of colour coding of doors and door furniture for residents and staff/service areas, aided cueing for residents.

Residents' rooms had a greater floor area than most case study homes visited, and the curved form of the main building allowed a variety of room shapes. The home had acknowledged that many people with dementia do not understand call systems, and research by the charity resulted in the use of a wireless system that offered a good facility for emergency calls by staff.

The general office and the manager's office were located near the main entrance, allowing discreet monitoring of the entrance area. Where appropriate, door security systems were fitted to safeguard residents.

Photograph 18: Clear personalised sign, but with an impersonal number

Views about Home F

Relatives

Liked the "smallness of the clusters".

Commented favourably on "the attention to detail and the homely environment".

Appreciated the "benefit of the town location with easy access to shops".

Managers and staff

"The tea kitchens attached to dining rooms are too small – could be the focal point for the group."

"Sluices should be in the centre of each cluster."

"The laundry could be more central – residents gather to watch."

"Access to garden considered to be important."

Although considered beneficial, "En suites are too small when using a wheelchair and two carers are involved".

"The importance of allowing adequate time for post-contract processes should be stressed."

"If there were no restrictions on site size, all accommodation would be on one floor with all residents having access to gardens."

Box 6.6: Design features – Home F

Enhancing features
- location of day rooms in centre of groups – minimises travel distances
- recessed fire doors (and sometimes radiators) eliminating potential obstructions and improving visual effect
- location of service plant in roof space
- attention to details which might confuse residents, including small items such as the omission of curtain holdbacks, fire 'break glass' points and finger plates
- mechanical extraction system.

Limiting features
- lack of parking areas near day rooms for wheelchairs or walking aids
- closed doors at the ends of corridors
- lack of shaving sockets and lights near mirrors in en suites.

Home G

As a result of a change of ownership, insufficient meaningful design information was available to enable us to provide full details here. We understand that the original client's brief had been firmly directed towards a nursing model based on a conventional hospital ward, and it was evident that little allowance had been made to reflect current knowledge of designing for people with dementia.

The first floor of the two-storey home was dedicated to dementia care and contained two wings of 15 residents' rooms linked symmetrically at each side of a central core block that contained day rooms, assisted bathrooms and WCs, and all other servicing facilities. The residents' rooms were arranged at either side of a straight corridor leading to a window, without a seat; the only variations being provided by recesses for the 15 entrance doors.

The original plan had located a nursing station centrally with views along the corridors of the residential wings and the corridor of the core block. However, when the new owners refurbished the home, the nursing station was removed and the central area was then used by residents as a popular meeting and sitting place.

Learning from practice: key messages

Box 6.7: Common issues

- There are mixed views about maintaining a separate and secure area for offices and service facilities with residents excluded. Some managers believe that, subject to health and safety controls, residents should have visual, if not physical, access to these areas and one manager spoke of residents standing at the door of the laundry watching the process – thoroughly investigate operational philosophy.
- Conduct thorough consultations with experienced staff on staff accommodation at design stage.
- Check that storage capacity in the laundry, including hanging facilities, adequately reflect the number of residents and the laundry regime.
- Innovative location of service equipment could release valuable floor space.
- Do not overlook storage for garden furniture.
- Consider providing adjoining residents' rooms which can be linked.
- Take care in choosing furniture in appropriate styles – although it may not be practicable to provide second-hand furniture from the relevant period, in most of the homes visited the furniture provided was in a modern style and did not recreate the familiarity of old wardrobes, drawers and cabinets.
- Introduce variety of style and height of seating in day rooms.
- Although involving additional cost, consider the benefit of a deeper sill, for ornaments, and a maximum height of 675mm above floor level; also ensure that transoms and controls do not impede the view.
- Research heating systems thoroughly.

7

Design consensus and debates

Introduction

This chapter draws on the literature and our case studies to discuss the main areas of consensus and debates in the design of care homes for people with dementia. It ends by considering some of the issues raised by the use of new technologies in care homes.

Consensus about 'best practice'

Design brief

Prior to the development of each home, a design brief was produced. In two cases it was developed in conjunction with the architect and – in one of these – the design and build contractor was also involved. The value of a comprehensive brief and thorough discussion involving experienced practitioners and designers was universally emphasised.

Location

The criteria for the ideal site were rarely met and compromises had to be made. In the case of the home on the edge-of-town site, the benefit of its location near to shopping and other local amenities outweighed the preference for a single-storey home. Other providers were attracted to a site either because it was owned by the relevant authority or a builder with appropriate experience, or it contained an outdated care home due for replacement. The options facing providers were limited, but in general the design solutions were successful.

First impressions

The following are important:

- Is it welcoming?
- Does the atmosphere 'feel good'?
- Is it cared for – well maintained, clean and fresh?
- Is the meaning of the layout clear? (Particularly important for people with dementia.)

Group living

All the homes had adopted a group-living model in design and care, although groups varied in size. In those with a group size of 15 or less, the day rooms, and in some cases service facilities, including bathrooms and WCs, were located centrally in the group. These arrangements created smaller, more or less symmetrical, secondary clusters of residents' rooms with resultant shorter travel distances for residents and staff.

Single-storey building

In practice, the decision to produce a design on one or two floors was dictated by the availability of a suitable site in the chosen area and the capital cost of building. Although the majority of providers and their staff would have favoured a single-storey home, the lack of a suitable site – in the right location linked with an affordable price per hectare – dictated that five out of seven were built as two-storey homes. *All* residents in the single-storey homes benefited from easy access to secure gardens, either outside the building footprint or within courtyards. Garden visits for those living at first-floor level were undoubtedly limited because of the time taken to travel to and from the garden.

Even residents able to walk to the garden unaided often needed assistance in the lift.

Wheelchair access

All homes were wheelchair user-friendly but few users were observed. Those who were, tended to be residents needing a wheelchair to move around the home but not for movement within their own rooms. However, 'barrier-free' features important to wheelchair users were intrinsic in the designs.

Residents' rooms

There were no shared rooms in the homes and all the homes would meet the new minimum standards[164] on resident rooms for 'existing single rooms'. Only a few rooms did not benefit from en suite facilities. The gross floor areas varied from 13.3 to 18m^2 per room and the effective usable bedroom floor space ranged from 10.8 to 12.4m^2. In the majority of homes the shape of the room maximised the usable floor area. However, where an entrance lobby had been created within the room, the effective usable space was reduced significantly. In only one such situation had a wardrobe been provided in the entrance area. The rooms without the limiting entrance lobby could maximise the floor area and provide more options for bed and other furniture positions.

Bed positions varied depending on the preferences of the residents or, if care needs prevailed, on the recommendation of staff to accommodate assistance with or without hoists or wheelchairs. There were instances in each home in which residents preferred a bed position away from the call system, ceiling light controls and electrical socket outlets. This highlighted the difficulty for designers in choosing favoured options for bed positions.

In order to allow space for residents' own familiar furniture, wardrobes had been fitted in only two homes and were reported as being too small. However, the opportunity to introduce their own was apparently not an option for many residents. As a consequence, bedroom furniture had been provided from standard modern low-cost ranges and created a bland uniformity not in keeping with one of the common criteria – to provide furniture in a style which would be familiar.

Corridors

Unless the group is small (that is, six or less) or the CADE approach, which arranges residents' rooms around a central area, is adopted, it is almost impossible to avoid corridors (depending on the definition of 'corridor'), but they can be shortened by careful planning.

In all but two of the homes visited, variable widths had been created in different ways with good results. In one instance, a recess wide enough to accommodate a couple of chairs and planters had been created, enhancing the corridor and providing another rest area.

Clean linen store

The need to have a clean linen store located in each group wing was commonly recognised, but the size of provision varied significantly – from 1.25m^2 for nine residents to 8.75m^2 serving 12 residents. When inadequate capacity was provided, other areas were brought into use. It was acknowledged that an adequate supply of clean linen in close proximity to the residents' rooms was beneficial and this also reduced the storage capacity required in the laundry.

Cleaning cupboard/store

The same comments apply to cleaning facilities. They should be adequate and easily accessed by staff when dealing with the consequences of accidents or spillage in group areas.

Utility and/or sluice room

These were all located on the group wings within easy reach of staff when dealing with routine daily situations. Homes had sluice rooms of varying size, some of which only had space to house the necessary equipment – bedpan washers, sluices – but two had space for dealing with soiled clothing and bedding, and useful benches.

Manager's office

In four homes, the manager's office was located near the entrance and near or adjoining the general office, which aided communication with administrative staff and visitors. In one home, the manager had an office on the first floor in a quieter zone but still retained a working desk in an office behind the general office. Some managers operated an 'open door' policy – open to staff and residents – others appeared to prefer to use it strictly for administration. This tended to reflect the management style of the home.

Staff accommodation

In most homes, the importance of providing generous space and suitable furnishings for staff had been observed, and in one home a dedicated outside terrace was available. The importance of suitable facilities to allow staff to relax away from residents was universally recognised but not always resolved satisfactorily. While it was not easy to calculate the space dedicated to each member of staff, when the figures were related to the number of residents, the allocation of space provided was reasonably consistent, ranging from 0.60 to 0.69m² per resident, with only one home falling below the range.

Two homes provided smoking and non-smoking rest rooms for staff although, in one of these, all staff tended to gather in the smoking room, leaving the non-smoking room unused. It was generally considered that rest rooms should be located close to the relevant working areas as staff were less inclined to use facilities if they were too far away, thus foregoing the opportunity to take important breaks in a stressful job.

Debates about 'best practice'

Day space

Which arrangement provides better opportunities for a wider range of activities: single living room combining sitting and dining areas, and perhaps a small kitchen area *or* separate rooms for sitting and dining with a small kitchen in the dining area or as a separate facility?

The single living room offers many benefits:

- a larger space for activities
- opportunity to vary allocation of space for various activities – achievable with furniture or screens
- easy visual contact between residents and staff, and consequently more effective use of staff time
- opportunity for residents' interests to be stimulated by association, for example, a resident in the sitting area could observe another engaged in an activity at a table in the dining area or in the kitchen area and be attracted to participate (Photograph 19)
- more possibility of the floor area being used efficiently through movement between the areas while still under the watchful eye of care staff
- a focal point of social and communal life for the group.

Photograph 19: Domestic activity as an attraction to other residents

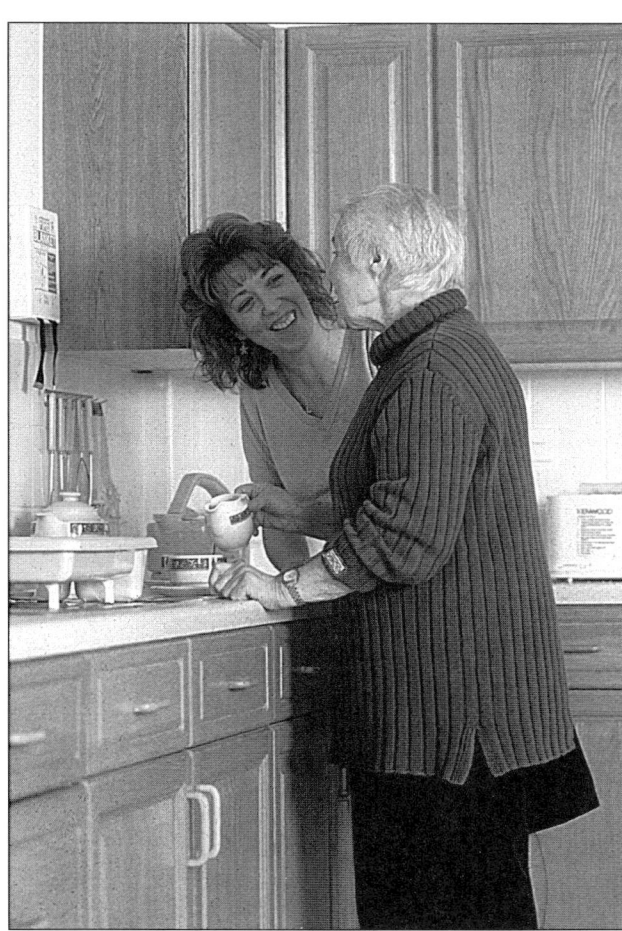

Separate sitting and dining rooms could produce other options:

- smaller rooms in which it should be easier to create a homely atmosphere
- in two homes dining rooms were also used for therapeutic activities, but this relied on the presence of a dedicated activities assistant
- it is easier to locate two separate rooms in the floor layout without disturbing the balance of resident groups, particularly if located at either side of the wing corridor.

Separate rooms, however, could create inefficient division of staff or, as was observed in some cases, could result in the dining room being used only at meal times. This could be further compounded when dining tables were laid immediately after one meal for the next, as residents were discouraged from disturbing the settings.

One issue about which there were mixed views was the location and use of the ubiquitous television set. On the one hand, it can be beneficial to have a set with a video recorder in a location where all or most of the residents in the group can gather. But, on the other, is the living room or the sitting room the best place? It is not uncommon to see television sets switched on regardless of the programme content or its suitability for residents. This can be distressing to residents seeking a quiet atmosphere. The solution appears to be a separate television room, although this use does not readily double as a quiet room. Another option is to have the television set located in the living room or sitting room, as it would in a family house, with a separate, genuine quiet room.

Residents' rooms

As long as there was sufficient space for care staff to deal with the needs of residents when using a hoist or wheelchair, without distress to either resident or staff, there was no complaint about the size of the room.

Relatives were more concerned than staff about the size of residents' rooms and their use as bed-sitting rooms. Operational managers generally considered that residents benefited from spending most of their waking time in an appropriate and stimulating environment in day rooms. Any proposal to increase the size of residents' rooms significantly would attract increased costs. In an ideal situation, care staff, managers, relatives and residents would welcome larger rooms so that the options for movement and personalisation could be increased.

En suite facilities

All homes provided en suite facilities. The provision of a shower within the facility, however, was still the subject of debate. Only one of the homes visited had showers in every en suite and, in another, only four en suites incorporated showers. Their use was limited and in only one instance was the resident able to manage without assistance. The majority view, however, was that showers should be provided in future homes.

In all cases, the door to the en suite opened into the bedroom area. In two cases, it was also fitted with 180° hinges allowing the door to open either way and, in one home, a secondary low intensity light in the WC provided a low source of illumination at night.

It was interesting to note that, whatever the floor area or dimensions of the en suite, care staff remarked that they had difficulty assisting residents when a hoist or wheelchair was involved. Even though the provision of a shower in the en suite created additional manoeuvring space, it was still important to ensure that sanitary ware did not impede staff when offering assistance.

Doors

Much has been written on the subject of the use of colours, both strong primary and pastel colours, and the embellishment with bells, knockers, numbers, name plates and frames for photographs or pictures. Of the case study homes, only two had used a range of strong colours and one, different pastel colours for each group wing, colour coded with decoration, carpets and soft furnishings. In the others, two had white painted and one wood veneer finishes to all residents' room doors.

The value of colour, door furniture and fittings was not always clear. In one case, the only reference point on the door was an anodised plate with space for a small name card and an engraved room number. The management and staff believed that the absence of clear visual cues on the door did not affect the ability of residents to locate their rooms successfully. On the other hand, general opinion was in favour of clear relevant cues, such as a familiar picture or photograph, supplemented by a large room number and a reasonable selection of familiar door furniture[165].

Central meeting area

In only one of the homes visited was there a dedicated area large enough to take all residents with carers. In one of the others, the home had been designed in such a way that, when coupled with the day centre and the adjoining reception area, it would accommodate most, if not all, residents and duty staff. Staff in the home with the large central area valued the facility for games, religious services, parties and dances. When not used in this way, it contained two or three small sitting areas in which residents could entertain guests or simply observe staff and visitors passing by. The addition of a furnished area to take all residents, however, could add significantly to the capital cost, whereas the creation of an appropriate area by combining day rooms, and/or day centre, with the entrance area produced an enterprising solution.

Quiet room

If residents, either individually or as a small group, wished to be in a quiet atmosphere, there was less possibility in one large dual-purpose living room. In some homes a small quiet room met this need.

Administration office

The location of this office varied. In three homes it was located adjacent to the reception area with outlook over the entrance. In addition, a desk in the reception area provided a focus for visitors and residents as well as, in one instance, a workstation for a volunteer employed for routine tasks.

Guest rooms

These featured in three homes although, in one, the room also doubled as an interview room. In another, where a twin guest room and a single room – which provided a sleep-over facility for staff – had been provided, there were plans to convert the facilities to resident rooms. The infrequency of use by relatives or friends did not justify the provision.

Whether or not there is a demand for guest rooms depends mainly on the location of the home, the proximity of suitable bed & breakfast accommodation and the domiciliary origins of residents. The more local the catchment area, the less likely the demand for guest accommodation will be.

Additional space requirements

In very simple terms: 'extra facilities = extra space = extra cost', unless duplication of space usage can be managed. This requires careful research into need before the design brief is finalised:

- Is a room needed for counselling relatives and staff?
- Are staff training courses to be held in the home?
- Do staff need quiet areas for administration or study?
- Is a meeting room required for medical or social care visitors?
- Is a separate handover room required? This will probably depend on the size of the home and the number of staff.
- Are nursing stations required?
- Is a treatment room required? This was provided in two case study homes (one nursing home and one residential home).

Use of technology

Technologies can be crudely divided into two as far as people with dementia are concerned – those which are for surveillance, monitoring and control ... and those which compensate for disability.
(Marshall, 1997, p 21[166])

Current applications of technology tend to relate to people, including some with dementia, still living in their own homes and whose needs relate more to issues of safety, such as movement or automatic cut-offs to cooker gas supply[167]. In such cases, equipment which has been demonstrated in 'smart homes' and subsequently used in numerous houses, is linked to a central control desk. The duty operator can then alert a relative, friend or, if necessary, summon help from a statutory body if assistance is required.

More sophisticated systems used in care homes in Australia are linked to a computer programme tailored to the care plan for the individual resident. In these cases, technology is not used to compensate for poor design or management, but primarily to provide more immediate monitoring, particularly through the night. It also allows staff to use time more effectively. The comprehensive system covers daytime security, night-time vigilance, and resident and staff management records. These records allow a more thorough analysis of resident movement and sleeping patterns, if required.

Many organisations are on the brink of using more advanced technology in care homes and some have made a tentative move, for example, by using sensors at skirting level to detect movement in a room. However, even though all the homes visited had incorporated, for example, induction loop systems, thermostatic blending valves to control water temperature at taps – and, in some cases, wireless call systems and electronic hold-open systems on fire doors – there was no evidence of more advanced technology.

8

Design recommendations

Introduction

The following recommendations, which should be associated with the previous chapter, emerge from the experience of management, staff, relatives, friends, residents and professional advisors of the homes visited – and the views of other specialists in the fields of designing, building or managing care homes for people with dementia. Notwithstanding the sources of the information, these recommendations are not directed towards any particular design model. It may be appropriate to provide a home 'under one roof' in a conventional style, or perhaps in the form of terraced housing, or may be in a series of linked houses or bungalows for groups of eight to ten residents – staffing requirements and financial feasibility will decide. The number of storeys in the building may be dictated either by site area or contours or by economic constraints. Similarly, the number of residents and size of group-living units will be determined by the provider, and will be strongly influenced by economic factors related to staffing provision and the proposed care regime.

Many good design features drawn from experience now regarded as standard good practice for residential and nursing care homes also hold good when designing for dementia care[168]. The following features, therefore, are either standard good practice features to be emphasised or important additional features specifically related to dementia care.

Size

Overall sizes of homes visited ranged from 24 to 72 places with group sizes varying from eight to 24 respectively. Generally, the larger the home overall and the larger the group, the more financially viable the home.

Assuming good occupancy rates, many factors are involved in determining financial viability. These factors include:

- cost-effective management of resources and services
- local authority fee structures
- number of self-funders
- local contractual arrangements.

Break-even for the homes visited occurred between home sizes of 36 and 60, and probably nearer the higher figure. One interviewee stated that: "a home would have to have 55 places to break even".

Different group sizes ranging from seven to fifteen, and secondary clusters of three to eight, operated with varying degrees of success. The optimal size, however, depends on the proposed overall capacity of the home resulting from a financial viability calculation, the staff:resident ratio and the physical constraints of the site.

In all but the largest home, the day rooms – and in some cases other relevant service facilities, such as assisted bathroom, linen store, utility room, and cleaners' cupboard – were located in the central core. The residents' rooms were separated into smaller sub-groups or clusters of three, four, five, six, seven or eight. Staff ratios of 1:4 or 1:5 existed and appeared to operate satisfactorily, with no significant difference arising from variation in size.

In the largest home of 72 places, the staff ratio was 1:8 – with cost savings, but with a noticeable increase in staff movement patterns, resulting not only from the reduced ratio but also from greater distances between the furthest resident and day rooms.

Location

Essential criteria relate to the catchment area, links with a strong local community and a good bus service, whether in an urban, suburban or rural setting. Increasingly, however, residents with advancing frailty become unable to walk from the home to visit local shops and other amenities and require transport. Distance from amenities is therefore less of a problem, although being located within the local community is a strong positive factor for the benefit of visiting relatives, friends and voluntary support.

Design concept

All the homes were 'under one roof' but the building footprints varied. It is for the architect to decide – with the owner – the most cost-effective shape within site constraints.

However, the design should be sensitive, domestic in scale and detail, and should create a base from which a homely effect can be produced. It should also:

- provide reasonable freedom of access to all low-risk areas, including gardens, ensuring that routes which may be used by inquisitive residents contain interesting features or suitable furniture
- provide a separate entrance for staff
- provide a number of small, semi-public sitting areas
- incorporate special points of interest to aid cueing for residents
- include features which enable opportunities for purposeful activities
- preclude situations which would allow invasive noise
- include domestic-style furniture, furnishings and fittings which will be familiar to residents
- minimise routine travel distances for staff
- allow for wheelchair access to all rooms used by residents
- make good use of natural and artificial lighting to avoid sharp contrasts, excessive brightness or dark, shadowed areas
- use different colour schemes for each group area
- ensure that views from residents' and day rooms are attractive
- ensure that the building is ergonomically and energy efficient.

Day care facilities

In two homes, day centres had been incorporated, each providing care for ten older people with a space allowance of 6/7m² per resident. These facilities not only provided links with the local community, but also acted as a source of potential long-term residents. In design terms, they were both located at the front of the home near the main entrance and provided an opportunity for alternative use when the day centre was not in operation. Such duplicated use could, if successfully managed as in the cases observed, improve the financial viability of the home.

Living areas

The various zones of a home within the building have been separated in this section into living areas, comprising primarily day spaces, and service areas, comprising areas mainly accessible only by staff, and the important features of each identified. These are followed by recommendations on furniture and furnishings, technology, and gardens and grounds.

Residents' rooms

Residents' rooms should have the following features:

- recessed entrance to allow personalisation with an A4 display panel – minimum – placed either on the door or beside it for a personal photograph or pictures, and the door fitted with domestic-style furniture

- minimum usable space, excluding the en suite, within a rectangular shape of 12m²
- window sills at a maximum height of 675mm above floor level
- two alternative positions for the bed with emergency system and light switch controls suitably located.

En suites

If a shower is provided, ensure that controls are located outside the range of the shower spray and that controls and handset can be operated from a seated position – a staff-operated cut-off valve should be fitted to water supplies. In addition, the following features should be provided:

- door with 180° hinges – helpful in an emergency
- adequate space for transfer from wheelchair or hoist, especially when two carers are needed
- view of WC from at least one preferred bed position
- structural provision for wall fixing of support rails

Photograph 20: Generous shelving for toiletries and personal supplies

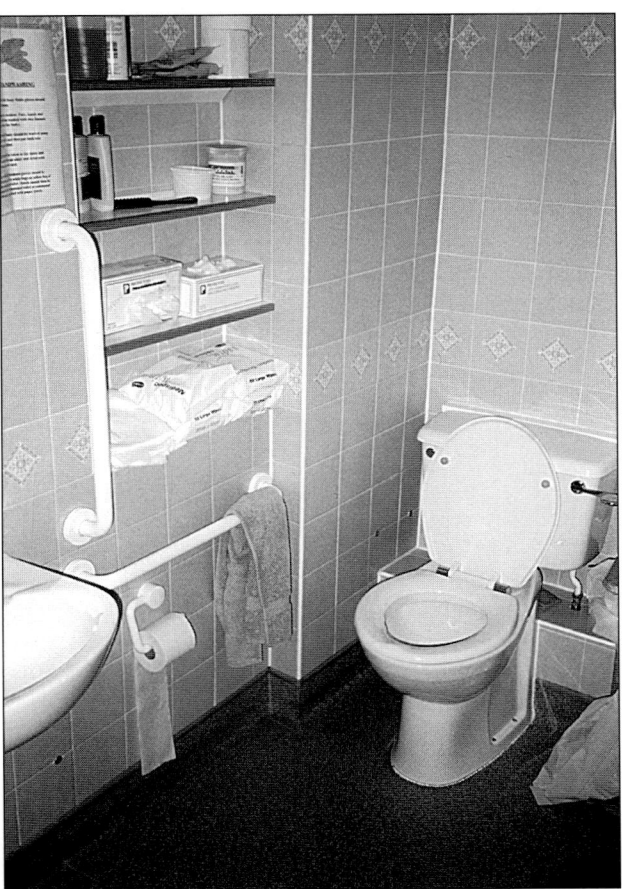

- practical shelving or other surface for toiletries within easy reach (Photograph 20)
- familiar, practical, sanitary fittings, such as bulbous capstan-style taps
- distinctive, contrasting colour, heavy-duty WC seat without cover – to withstand heavy impact
- toilet roll holder within easy reach of WC
- matt finishes to wall and floor coverings.

Sitting room and dining room or combined living room

The choice of arrangement will depend on the care practices to be operated in the home but the area per resident should be above registration standards at about 6m² and should:

- be located centrally in the wing with well lit approaches
- provide widened door openings and glazed doors and/or panels to corridor walls to allow approaching residents a clear and early view into the room
- have attractive, easy access to gardens when at ground-floor level
- have a system of lighting which can be controlled to provide suitable levels of illumination for a range of activities from sitting and relaxing to reading.

Quiet room (if provided)

The floor area should be no greater than 20m² to preserve domestic scale. It may be shared between groups and should be:

- near the main day rooms and furnished in a homely style which will be familiar to residents.

Corridors

These always have an important role in care homes and should:

- be as attractive and short as possible, and provide cueing features or opportunities
- benefit from natural light, with appropriate intensity of artificial light, and suitable ventilation
- not contain tempting 'no-go' areas, for example, behind locked glazed doors.

They should have:

- a minimum width of 1500mm
- variation in width utilising areas created by recessed entrances
- entrance doors to residents' rooms set in recesses and arranged so that they do not face across the corridor
- handrails on both sides with protrusions or grooves near the ends, as an aid to visually impaired people
- recessed settings for radiators and fire doors, which should be fitted with 'hold open' door closers
- a sitting area with a view at any outer end to avoid a closed door or cul-de-sac effect
- doors to staff-only areas coloured to blend with adjoining walls.

Meeting area

The most cost-effective means of providing a meeting area to accommodate all, or most, residents and duty staff, is to combine rooms for other purposes with the entrance area. If a day centre is included at the home this also may form part of the main area. The need for this area will depend on several factors, including the planned care practices and overall financial viability. If provided, the cumulative space allowance should be approximately 4m² per resident.

Activity room

Ideally a separate room for therapeutic activities should be provided, with a dedicated assistant. Some homes, however, utilise dining rooms or dining areas of living rooms.

Assisted bathrooms

Should include:

- matt finishes to wall and floor coverings
- a level-access shower with controls outside the immediate shower area and slide adjustable handset conveniently positioned for operation from an independent seat
- a user-friendly specialist bath suitable for independent and assisted use (Photographs 21a, b and c)
- light switches inside to avoid interference by passers-by
- a door with a distinctive colour and clear pictorial sign
- natural light, if possible
- there is no reason why sanitary ware should not be coloured.

Photographs 21a-c: Are *all* these baths user friendly?

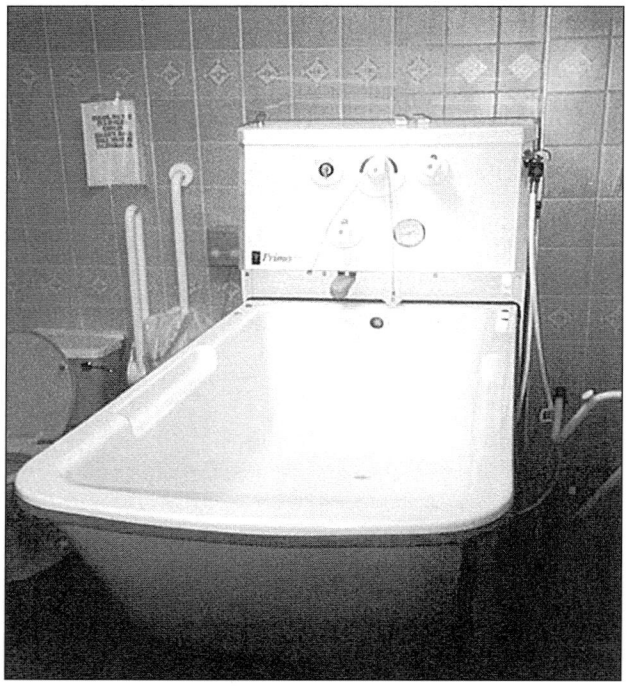
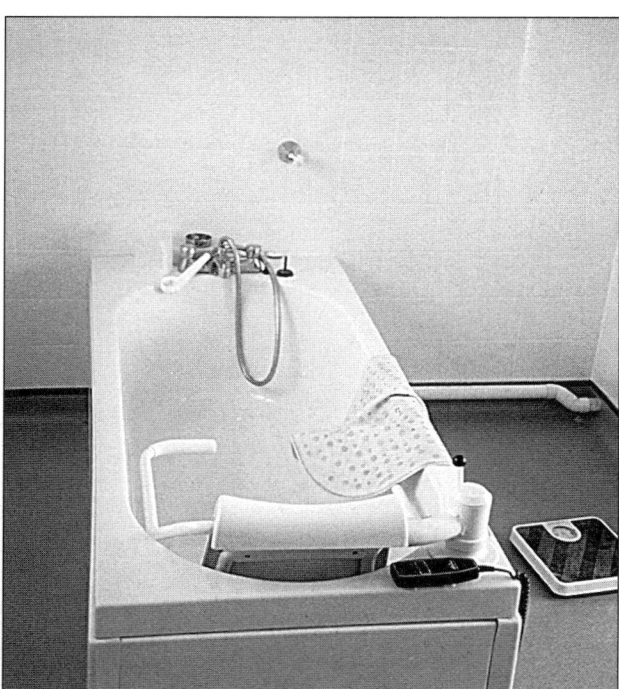

Design recommendations

Assisted WC

- this should meet disabled and assisted standards, be in close proximity to the day rooms and clearly identified (Photograph 22)
- again there is no reason why sanitary ware should not be coloured.

Photograph 22: Clear sign, but check the recognition factor

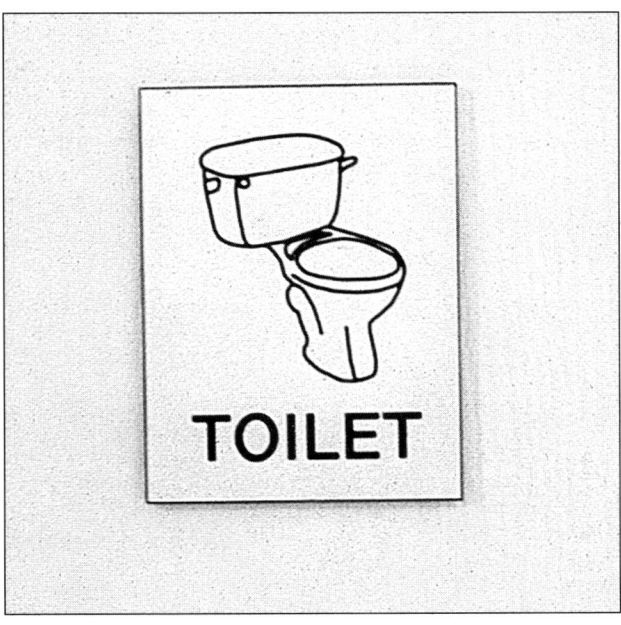

Photograph 21c

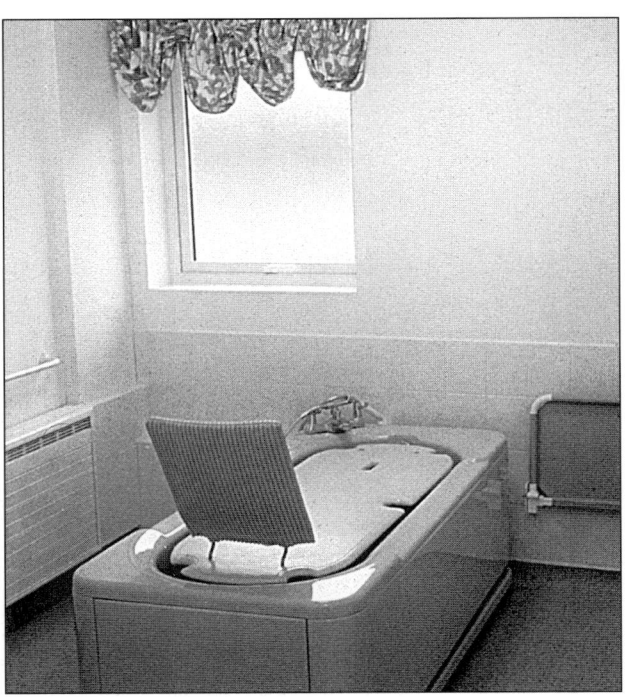

Service areas

Service areas relevant to the needs of each resident group should be provided within the group area and be separated from the main service facilities for the home, such as kitchen, laundry and general storage.

Group facilities

Facilities for each group should be located in a convenient position, bearing in mind the greater likelihood of accidents and continence problems. The 'clean and cleaning' facilities could be grouped together:

- linen store with sufficient capacity to cope with the number of residents in the group
- cleaning cupboard with a draining board and deep sink and storage for cleaning equipment and materials
- utility room incorporating bed-pan washer and deep sink, worktop/draining board and wash hand basin
- depending on the number of bathrooms required, they could be located either at the outer limits of the group area or in a central position, but positioned so that no resident has an unnecessarily long walk.

General storage

This is a standard requirement but ensure that adequate capacity is provided.

Room for handover, training and/or counselling

Management needs to decide on need, size and affordability. Many staff, however, believe that a training room in a dementia care home is important.

Kitchen

A specialist design is advised but ensure adequate parking for heated trolleys, if they are required.

Laundry

Provide adequate shelf and hanging space for clean laundry and floor space for laundry trolleys to reflect the increased workload (check the laundry system proposed first).

Staff accommodation

Provide comfortable, well-equipped rest room(s), preferably not too far from group areas.

Furniture and furnishings

Endeavour to create familiar styles with:

- lounge seating in a variety of styles and covers including settees, but ensure that an appropriate seat height is produced[169]
- a high percentage of dining chairs with arms which extend over the front legs to provide stable leverage support when leaving the chair
- tables for six – preferably circular
- no abrupt changes in colour and/or pattern in floor coverings.

Technology

Even if there is no immediate intention to invest in 'advanced technology', at the very least hardwiring or accessible cable conduits should be routed to each room and linked with the general office or prospective control base. This would increase future options for the connection of relevant and suitable equipment.

Gardens and grounds

The aim should be to provide safe, secure, interesting and accessible areas with high quality hard and soft landscaping, incorporating suitable surfaces and planting to take into account the impairments that residents may experience. Trees and large shrubs should not overhang footpaths, which should be in view from the home and not screened by buildings, trees or shrubberies. Raised beds and sheltered sitting areas should be provided, but low walls should be avoided. Familiar garden objects such as wooden seats, bird tables, sheds and greenhouses all enhance the outdoor environment.

9

Conclusion

Our knowledge about how best to design and manage care homes for people with dementia has advanced significantly. There is still much to learn. This book concludes that while the principles of good practice are clear, there is no single 'right' way to design and manage specialist dementia care homes. Decisions about design, the model of service and economic viability need to be considered in tandem. With current standard revenue funding, providers of specialist dementia care homes have to compromise in combining the implementation of best practice principles and achievement of financial viability.

This report provides a great deal of detailed advice about management, care practice, staffing, and building design for specialist dementia care homes. In summary, it recommends that in setting up or developing high quality care homes for people with dementia, providers should:

- set out with, and maintain, a commitment to excellence in dementia care
- ensure plans match local needs; and that the planning work involved is not underestimated
- develop the service model and building design in tandem, applying the principles and features of best practice to local requirements and circumstances
- choose a site with access to community facilities and good public transport
- invest in good design; this benefits residents, staff and the business
- ensure the building designer will produce to requirements, on time and within budget; agree essential features before finalising the design
- attend to the design details; they enhance the quality of life for people with dementia
- manage the opening of a new home as a project in itself
- invest in recruiting the best possible home manager with the knowledge, experience, skills, leadership qualities and commitment for the job
- ensure that managers and staff are equipped to implement best practice ideas in person-centred dementia care
- enhance staffing levels to provide residents with the individualised attention that is central to person-centred dementia care
- carefully select, train, support, value and involve all staff; the importance of good staff management cannot be overestimated
- develop ways to involve relatives and residents with dementia in influencing individual care and the management of the home
- enhance the residents' care and quality of life through good links with local health and social care services, community groups and other local resources.

We conclude with the words of a member of our project Advisory Group:

"You cannot separate out good design, effective management and user involvement for people with dementia. If you do, you're left with bricks and mortar, sterile consultancy-speak or nodding platitudes. It's only when you take the three together that you demonstrate that you're serious about making a difference." (Alex O'Neil, Joseph Rowntree Foundation)

End notes

Preface

1. DoH (Department of Health) (1998) *Modernising social services: Promoting independence, improving protection raising standards*, Cm 4169, London: The Stationery Office.

    DoH (2001a) *Care homes for older people: National minimum standards*, London: The Stationery Office.

    DoH (2001b) *National service framework for older people*, London: DoH.

    Care Standards Act 2000, London: The Stationery Office.

    Human Rights Act 1998, London: The Stationery Office.

    Health Service Act 2001 (Care Homes), London: The Stationery Office.

2. Laing, W. (1998) *A fair price for care? Disparities between market rates for nursing/residential care and what state funding agencies will pay*, York: York Publishing Services.

    Andrews, G.A. and Phillips, D.R. (2000) 'Moral dilemmas and the management of private residential homes: the impact of care in the community reforms in the UK', *Ageing and Society*, vol 20, no 5, pp 599-622.

3. Johnson, M.L., Cullen, L. and Patsios, D. (1999) *Managers in long-term care: Their quality and qualities*, Bristol/York: The Policy Press/Joseph Rowntree Foundation.

    Office of Fair Trading (1998) *Older people as consumers in care homes: A report by the Office of Fair Trading*, OFT No 242, London: Office of Fair Trading.

4. Based on:
    DoH (2000) 'Community care statistics: residential personal social services for adults, England', Bulletin 2000/28, London: DoH.

    DoH (2001c) 'Community care statistics: private nursing homes, hospitals and clinics', Bulletin 2001/7, London: DoH.

5. National Institute for Social Work (1997) *Measuring the quality of residential care*, Briefing No 21, London: National Institute for Social Work.

6. Based on a total of approximately 240,300 people aged 65+ in residential homes. From:
    DoH (2000) 'Community care statistics: residential personal social services for adults, England', Bulletin 2000/28, London: DoH.

7. Alzheimer Scotland – Action on Dementia (2000) *Planning signposts for dementia care services*, Edinburgh: Alzheimer Scotland – Action on Dementia.

8. Bartlett, H. and Burnip, S. (1999) 'Improving care in nursing and residential homes', *Generations Review*, vol 9, no 1, pp 8-10.

9. DoH (2001b) *National service framework for older people*, London: DoH.

10. Kellaher, L. (1998) 'When and how institutions do work – the Caring in Homes Initiative', in R. Jack (ed) *Residential versus community care: The role of institutions in welfare provision*, Basingstoke: Macmillan, pp 185-201.

[11] Mozley, C.G., Huxley, P., Sutcliffe, C., Bagley, H., Burns, A., Challis, D. and Cordingley, L. (1999) 'Not knowing where I am doesn't mean I don't know what I like: cognitive impairment and quality of life responses in elderly people', *International Journal of Geriatric Psychiatry*, vol 14, no 9, pp 776-83.

Allan, K. (2001) *Communication and consultation: Exploring ways for staff to involve people with dementia in developing services*, Bristol/York: The Policy Press/Joseph Rowntree Foundation.

Chapter 1: First steps in planning and establishing a dementia care home

Establishing values and principles

[12] DoH/Social Services Inspectorate (1993) *Standards for the residential care of elderly people with mental disorders*, Inspecting for Quality Series, London: HMSO.

CPA (Centre for Policy on Ageing) (1996) *A better home life: A code of good practice for residential and nursing home care*, Advisory Group convened by Centre for Policy on Ageing, Chaired by Kina, Lady Avebury, London: CPA.

[13] King's Fund (1986) *Living well into old age: Applying principles of good practice to services for people with dementia – project paper*, London: King's Fund Publishing Office.

[14] Cox, S., Anderson, I., Dick, S. and Elgar, J. (1998) *The person, the community and dementia: Developing a value framework*, Stirling: Dementia Services Development Centre.

Providing what people with dementia and their relatives want

[15] Bamford, C. and Bruce, E. (2000) 'Defining the outcomes of community care: the perspectives of older people with dementia and their carers', *Ageing and Society*, vol 20, no 5, pp 543-70.

Allan, K. (2001) *Communication and consultation: Exploring ways for staff to involve people with dementia in developing services*, Bristol/York: The Policy Press/Joseph Rowntree Foundation.

[16] Counsel and Care (1992a) *From home to a home*, Forward by Lady Howe, London: Counsel and Care.

Raynes, N. (1999) 'Older residents' participation in specifying quality in nursing and residential care homes', *Generations Review*, vol 9, no 2, pp 10-12.

Challiner, Y. (2000) 'The "Ideal Home" study: seeking consumers' views in elderly long-term care', *Generations Review*, vol 10, no 2, pp 8-10.

Kellaher, L. (2000) *A choice well made: Mutuality as a governing principle in residential care*, London: CPA.

[17] See also:
Morgan, D.G. and Stewart, N.J. (1999) 'The physical environment of special care units: needs of residents with dementia from the perspective of staff and family caregivers', *Qualitative Health Research*, vol 9, no 1, pp 105-18.

Deciding on a service model

[18] *Care Standards Act 2000*, Chapter 14, London: The Stationery Office.

[19] Netten, A. (1993) *A positive environment? Physical and social influences on people with senile dementia in residential care*, Aldershot/Canterbury: Ashgate/Personal Social Services Research Unit, University of Kent.

[20] Allister, C.L. and Silverman, M.A. (1999) 'Community formation and community roles among persons with Alzheimer's disease: a comparative study of experience in a residential Alzheimer's facility and a traditional nursing home', *Qualitative Health Research*, vol 9, no 1, pp 65-8.

[21] Tooth, J. (1996) 'Who wants a home for life?', *Journal of Dementia Care*, vol 4, no 4, pp 12-14.

[22] Wilkin, D. (1986) 'The mix of lucid and confused residents', in K. Judge and I. Sinclair (eds) *Residential care for elderly people*, London: HMSO, pp 183-9.

Willcocks, D., Peace, S. and Kellaher, L. (1987) *Private lives in public places: A research-based critique of residential life in local authority old people's homes*, London: Tavistock Publications.

Fahrenfort, M. (1997) 'In search of the best environment: results of five experiments in the institutional organisation of care for demented people', in B.M.L. Miesen and G.M.M. Jones (eds) *Care-giving in dementia: Research and applications, Vol 2*, London: Routledge, pp 287-301.

Reed, J. (1999) 'Keeping a distance: the reactions of older people in care homes to confused fellow residents', in T. Adams and C. Clarke (eds) *Dementia care: Developing partnerships in practice*, London: Bailliere Tindall, pp 165-86.

[23] Wilkin, D. (1986) 'The mix of lucid and confused residents', in K. Judge and I. Sinclair (eds) *Residential care for elderly people*, London: HMSO, pp 183-9.

[24] Marshall, M. (1993) *Small scale, domestic style, longstay accommodation for people with dementia*, Stirling: Dementia Services Development Centre.

Tester, S. (1999) *The quality challenge: Caring for people with dementia in residential institutions in Europe*, Edinburgh: Alzheimer Scotland – Action on Dementia.

[25] Marshall, M. (1993) *Small scale, domestic style, longstay accommodation for people with dementia*, Stirling: Dementia Services Development Centre.

[26] Alzheimer Scotland – Action on Dementia (2000) *Planning signposts for dementia care services*, Edinburgh: Alzheimer Scotland – Action on Dementia.

Peace, S., Kellaher, L. and Willcocks, D. (1997) *Re-evaluating residential care*, Rethinking Ageing Series, Buckingham: Open University Press.

Marshall, M. (1998) 'Therapeutic buildings for people with dementia', in S. Judd, M. Marshall and P. Phippen (eds) *Design for dementia*, London: Hawker Publications, pp 11-14.

[27] Alzheimer Scotland – Action on Dementia (2000) *Planning signposts for dementia care services*, Edinburgh: Alzheimer Scotland – Action on Dementia.

[28] Netten, A. (1993) *A positive environment? Physical and social influences on people with senile dementia in residential care*, Aldershot/Canterbury: Ashgate/Personal Social Services Research Unit, University of Kent.

Mountain, G. and Godfrey, M. (1995) *Respite care provision for older people with dementia: A review of the literature*, Leeds: Nuffield Institute for Health, University of Leeds.

[29] Moriarty, J. and Webb, S. (2000) *Part of their lives: Community care for older people with dementia*, Bristol: The Policy Press.

[30] Cunningham, G. and Dick, S. (1995) *More than just a break: A study of carers' views about respite care services for people with dementia*, Edinburgh: Alzheimer Scotland – Action on Dementia.

Mountain, G. and Godfrey, M. (1995) *Respite care provision for older people with dementia: A review of the literature*, Leeds: Nuffield Institute for Health, University of Leeds.

Moriarty, J. and Levin, E. (1998) 'Respite care in homes and hospitals', in R. Jack (ed) *Residential versus community care: The role of institutions in welfare provision*, Basingstoke: Macmillan, pp 124-39.

Briggs, K. and Askham, J. (1999) *Needs of people with dementia and those who care for them – A review of the literature*, London: Alzheimer's Society.

Counsel and Care (1995) *Last nights*, London: Counsel and Care.

Deciding on the resident group

[31] Kellaher, L. (2000) *A choice well made: Mutuality as a governing principle in residential care*, London: CPA.

[32] Audit Commission (2000) *Forget me not: Mental health services for older people*, London: Audit Commission.

[33] Challis, D., Carpenter, I. and Traske, K. (1996) *Assessment in continuing care homes: Towards a national standard instrument*, Canterbury: Personal Social Services Research Unit, University of Kent.

Providing for residents with specific needs

[34] See for example:
Cox, S. and Keady, J. (eds) (1999) *Younger people with dementia: Planning, practice, and development*, London: Jessica Kingsley Publishers.

[35] Patel, N., Mirza, N.R., Lindblad, P., Armstrup, K. and Samaoli, O. (1998) *Dementia and minority ethnic older people: Managing care in the UK, Denmark and France*, Lyme Regis: Russell House Publishing.

For general guidance on caring for older people from ethnic minority communities see:
Alibhai-Brown, Y. (1998) *Caring for ethnic minority elders*, London: Age Concern.

[36] Cox, S. (1998) *Home solutions: Housing and support for people with dementia*, London: HACT.

[37] Jones, A., Marcia, P. and Maynard, C. (1992) *A home from home: The experience of black residential projects as a focus of good practice*, London: National Institute for Social Work.

Relocation

[38] Review Panel, Stephen Farrow (Chair) (1997) *Report of the review panel into the deaths of eight patients following their transfer from Napsbury Hospital to Elmstead House Nursing Home*, the Review Panel, consisting of the following organisations: Age Concern England, Barnet Health Authority, Barnet Healthcare Trust, Barnet Local Medical Committee, Community Health Services Ltd, London Borough of Barnet, London: Barnet Health Authority.

Chapter 2: Management matters

[39] Gilloran, A. and Downs, M. (1997) 'Issues of staffing and therapeutic care', in S. Hunter (ed) *Dementia challenges and new directions*, Research Highlights in Social Work No 31, London: Jessica Kingsley Publishers, pp 165-81.

Kitwood, T. and Woods, B. (1996) *Training and development strategy for dementia care in residential settings*, Bradford: Bradford Dementia Group.

[40] Schneider, J., Mann, A., Blizard, B. and Kharicha, K. (1997) *Quality of residential care for elderly people phase II study extension*, Discussion Paper No 1304, Canterbury: Personal Social Services Research Unit, University of Kent.

[41] Herbert, G. (1997) 'What hat should we wear today? Recruiting and developing the ideal workforce for dementia care', in M. Marshall (ed) *State of the art in dementia care*, London: CPA, pp 111-15.

Recruitment and selection

[42] Johnson, M.L., Cullen, L. and Patsios, D. (1999) *Managers in long-term care: Their quality and qualities*, Bristol/York: The Policy Press/Joseph Rowntree Foundation.

[43] Ford, P. and Heath, H. (eds) (1996) *Nursing homes: Nursing values*, London: Royal College of Nursing.

[44] Johnson, M.L., Cullen, L. and Patsios, D. (1999) *Managers in long-term care: Their quality and qualities*, Bristol/York: The Policy Press/Joseph Rowntree Foundation.

[45] Redfern, S.J. (1998) 'Is there still a role for nursing?', in R. Jack (ed) *Residential versus community care*, Basingstoke: Macmillan, pp 166-84.

[46] Alzheimer's Society (2000) *Alzheimer's Society response: Fit for the Future? National required standards for residential and nursing homes for older people*, London: Alzheimer's Society.

[47] Johnson, M.L., Cullen, L. and Patsios, D. (1999) *Managers in long-term care: Their quality and qualities*, Bristol/York: The Policy Press/Joseph Rowntree Foundation.

Good leadership

[48] Mattiasson, A. and Andersson, L. (1995) 'Organisational environment and the support of patient autonomy in nursing home care', *Journal of Advanced Nursing*, vol 22, pp 1149-57.

[49] Gilloran, A., Robertson, A., McGlew, T. and McKee, K. (1995) 'Improving work satisfaction amongst nursing staff and quality of care for elderly patients with dementia: some policy implications', *Ageing and Society*, vol 15, no 3, pp 375-91.

Kitwood, T., Buckland, S. and Petre, T. (1995) *Brighter futures: A report on research into provision for persons with dementia in residential homes, nursing homes and sheltered housing*, Kidlington: Anchor Housing Association.

[50] Gilloran, A., Robertson, A., McGlew, T. and McKee, K. (1995) 'Improving work satisfaction amongst nursing staff and quality of care for elderly patients with dementia: some policy implications', *Ageing and Society*, vol 15, no 3, pp 375-91.

[51] Kitwood, T., Buckland, S. and Petre, T. (1995) *Brighter futures: A report on research into provision for persons with dementia in residential homes, nursing homes and sheltered housing*, Kidlington: Anchor Housing Association.

[52] Gilloran, A., Robertson, A., McGlew, T. and McKee, K. (1995) 'Improving work satisfaction amongst nursing staff and quality of care for elderly patients with dementia: some policy implications', *Ageing and Society*, vol 15, no 3, pp 375-91.

[53] Eastman, M. (1998) 'Why and when institutions do not work – *Sans everything* revisited', in R. Jack (ed) *Residential versus community care: The role of institutions in welfare provision*, Basingstoke: Macmillan.

Burton, J. (1998) *Managing residential care*, London: Routledge.

Quality management

[54] DoH (2001a) *Care homes for older people: National minimum standards*, London: The Stationery Office.

[55] Johnson, M.L., Cullen, L. and Patsios, D. (1999) *Managers in long-term care: Their quality and qualities*, Bristol/York: The Policy Press/Joseph Rowntree Foundation.

[56] Challiner, Y. (1997) 'Introducing quality assurance into long term care for elderly people: a difficult and worthwhile process?', *Quality in Health Care*, vol 6, pp 153-9.

[57] Murphy, E., Lindesay, J. and Dean, R. (1994) *The Domus project: Long term care for older people with dementia*, London: Sainsbury Centre for Mental Health.

Perrin, T. (1997) 'Occupational need in severe dementia: a descriptive study', *Journal of Advanced Nursing*, no 25, pp 934-41.

[58] Bradford Dementia Group (1997) *Evaluating dementia care: the DCM method*, 7th edn, Bradford: University of Bradford.

Perrin, T. (1997) 'Occupational need in severe dementia: a descriptive study', *Journal of Advanced Nursing*, no 25, pp 934-41.

[59] Alzheimer's Society and Royal College of Nursing (2001) *Quality dementia care in care homes: Person centred standards*, London: Alzheimer's Society.

[60] O'Kell, S. (1995) *Care standards in the residential care sector*, York: York Publishing Services.

[61] Cox, S. (2001) 'Developing quality in services', in C. Cantley (ed) *A handbook of dementia care*, Buckingham: Open University Press.

[62] Bradford Dementia Group (1997) *Evaluating dementia care: The DCM method*, 7th edn, Bradford: University of Bradford.

End notes

Staff management

63 Jaques, A. and Innes, A. (1998) 'Who cares about care assistant work?', *Journal of Dementia Care*, vol 6, no 6, pp 33-7.

64 Workman, B.A. (1996) 'An investigation into how the health care assistants perceive their role as "support workers" to the qualified staff', *Journal of Advanced Nursing*, vol 23, no 3, pp 612-19.

65 Kitwood, T. and Woods, B. (1996) *Training and development strategy for dementia care in residential settings*, Bradford: Bradford Dementia Group.

Involving relatives and residents

66 Abbott, S., Fisk, M. and Forward, L. (2000) 'Social and democratic participation in residential settings for older people: realities and aspirations', *Ageing and Society*, vol 20, no 3, pp 327-40.

67 Counsel and Care (1992a) *From home to a home*, Forward by Lady Howe, London: Counsel and Care.

68 Allan, K. (2001) *Communication and consultation: Exploring ways for staff to involve people with dementia in developing services*, Bristol/York: The Policy Press/Joseph Rowntree Foundation.

External services

69 Royal College of Physicians (2000) *The health and care of older people in care homes*, A report of a joint working party of the Royal College of Physicians, Royal College of Nursing and British Geriatrics Society, London: Royal College of Physicians.

Avards, R., Bright, L. and Davies, S. (1998) *Bringing health to homes*, London: Counsel and Care.

Management development

70 Johnson, M.L., Cullen, L. and Patsios, D. (1999) *Managers in long-term care: Their quality and qualities*, Bristol/York: The Policy Press/Joseph Rowntree Foundation.

Chapter 3: Care matters

71 Chapman, A., Jaques, A. and Marshall, M. (1994) *Dementia care: A handbook for residential and day care*, London: Age Concern England.

Holden, U. and Woods, R.T. (1995) *Positive approaches to dementia care*, 3rd edn, London: Churchill Livingstone.

Phair, L. and Good, V. (1998) *Dementia – a positive approach*, London: Whurr Publishers.

Garratt, S. and Hamilton-Smith, E. (1995) *Rethinking dementia: An Australian approach*, Melbourne: Ausmed.

Person-centred care

72 Perrin, T. (1997) 'Occupational need in severe dementia: a descriptive study', *Journal of Advanced Nursing*, no 25, pp 934-41.

73 Crisp, J. (1999) 'Towards a partnership in maintaining personhood', in T. Adams and C. Clarke (eds) *Dementia care: Developing partnerships in practice*, London: Bailliere Tindall, pp 95-119.

74 Murphy, C. (1994) *"It started with a sea shell": Life story work and people with dementia*, Stirling: Dementia Services Development Centre.

75 Kitwood, T., Buckland, S. and Petre, T. (1995) *Brighter futures: A report on research into provision for persons with dementia in residential homes, nursing homes and sheltered housing*, Kidlington: Anchor Housing Association.

Communication

76 Goldsmith, M. (1996) *Hearing the voice of people with dementia: Opportunities and obstacles*, London: Jessica Kingsley Publishers.

Killick, J. and Allan, K. (2001) *Communication and the care of people with dementia*, Buckingham: Open University Press.

Innes, A. and Capstick, A. (2001) 'Communication and personhood', in C. Cantley (ed) *A handbook of dementia care*, Buckingham: Open University Press.

[77] Goldsmith, M., Kindred, M. and Innes, A. (1997) *Hearing the voice of people with dementia: A study guide for care staff and volunteers who work with people with dementia*, Stirling: Dementia Services Development Centre.

Clarke, A., Hollands, J. and Smith, J. (1996) *Windows to a damaged world*, London: Counsel and Care.

Powell, J. (2000) *Care to communicate: Helping the older person with dementia*, London: Hawker Publications.

Killick, J. and Allan, K. (2001) *Communication and the care of people with dementia*, Buckingham: Open University Press.

'Challenging' behaviour

[78] Moniz-Cook, E., Woods, R. and Gardiner, E. (2000) 'Staff factors associated with perception of behaviour as "challenging" in residential and nursing homes', *Aging and Mental Health*, vol 4, no 1, pp 48-55.

[79] Innes, A. (1998) 'Behind labels: what makes behaviour "difficult"', *Journal of Dementia Care*, vol 6, no 5, pp 22-5.

[80] For example:
Stokes, G. (2000) *Challenging behaviour*, Bicester: Winslow Press.

[81] For a training guide on managing 'challenging' behaviour see, for example:
Chapman, A., Jackson, G.A. and McDonald, C. (1999) *What behaviour? Whose problem?*, Stirling: Dementia Services Development Centre.

[82] Moniz-Cook, E., Agar, S., Silver, M., Woods, R., Wang, M., Elston, C. and Win, T. (1998) 'Can staff training reduce behavioural problems in residential care for the elderly mentally ill?', *International Journal of Geriatric Psychiatry*, vol 13, no 3, pp 149-58.

Spirituality and sexuality

[83] Sherman, B. (1999) *Sex, intimacy, and aged care*, London: Jessica Kingsley Publishers.

Howse, K. (1999) *Religion, spirituality and older people*, CPA Report No 25, London: CPA.

Jewell, A. (ed) (1999) *Spirituality and ageing*, London: Jessica Kingsley Publishers.

[84] Archibald, C. (1994) 'Sex: is it a problem?', *Journal of Dementia Care*, vol 2, no 4, pp 16-17.

Archibald, C. (1998) 'Sexuality, dementia and residential care: managers report and response', *Health and Social Care in the Community*, vol 6, no 2, pp 95-101.

[85] Regan, D. and Smith, J. (1997) *The fullness of time: How homes for older people can respond to their residents' need for wholeness and a spiritual dimension to care*, London: Counsel and Care.

[86] Moffitt, L. (1996) 'Helping to re-create a personal sacred space', *Journal of Dementia Care*, vol 4, no 3, pp 19-21.

Care planning

[87] Office of Fair Trading (1998) *Older people as consumers in care homes: A report by the Office of Fair Trading*, OFT No 242, London: Office of Fair Trading.

CPA (Centre for Policy on Ageing) (1996) *A better home life: A code of good practice for residential and nursing home care*, Advisory Group convened by Centre for Policy on Ageing, Chaired by Kina, Lady Avebury, London: CPA.

Clarke, A., Hollands, J. and Smith, J. (1996) *Windows to a damaged world*, London: Counsel and Care.

[88] Mallinson, I. (1996) *Care planning in residential care for older people in Scotland*, Aldershot: Avebury.

Coleman, V., Regan, D. and Smith, J. (1999) *Who cares plans: A guide to care planning in homes for older people*, London: Counsel and Care.

[89] Smith, M. and Cantley, C. (in preparation) *Report on an action research project to develop care planning for people with dementia in care homes*, Newcastle upon Tyne: Dementia North, University of Northumbria.

[90] Foster, K. (1997) 'Pragmatic groups: interactions and relationships between people with dementia', in M. Marshall (ed) *State of the art in dementia care*, London: CPA, pp 57-62.

[91] O'Donovan, S. (1994) *Simon's nursing assessment manual: For the care of older people with dementia*, Bicester: Winslow Press Ltd.

Oyebode, J., Evans, A., Foster, N., McDermott, P. and Pyke, P. (1996) 'Creating a new, individualised service', *Journal of Dementia Care*, vol 4, no 5, pp 18-19.

[92] Fleming, R., Bowles, J., Todd, S. and Kramer, T. (Staff of Sinclair Home) (1996) *Model care plans for carers of people with dementia*, Sydney, Australia: The Hammond Care Group.

[93] Garratt, S. and Hamilton-Smith, E. (1995) *Rethinking dementia: An Australian approach*, Melbourne: Ausmed.

[94] Coleman, V., Regan, D. and Smith, J. (1999) *Who cares plans: A guide to care planning in homes for older people*, London: Counsel and Care.

Therapies and activities

[95] Brooker, D. (2001) 'Therapeutic activity', in C. Cantley (ed) *A handbook of dementia care*, Buckingham: Open University Press.

[96] For use of aromatherapy in dementia care see, for example:
Burleigh, S. and Armstrong, C. (1997) 'On the scent of a useful therapy', *Journal of Dementia Care*, vol 5, no 4, pp 21-3.

Kirkpatrick, J. and Wood, J. (1998) 'Aromatherpy's benefits', *Journal of Dementia Care*, vol 6, no 3, p 9.

[97] Gibson, F. (1998) *Reminiscence and recall*, 2nd edn, London: Age Concern England.

Gibson, F. (1994) 'What can reminiscence contribute to people with dementia?', in J. Bornat (ed) *Reminiscence reviewed: Evaluations, achievements, perspectives*, Buckingham: Open University Press.

[98] Feil, N. (1993) *The validation breakthrough: Simple techniques for communicating with people with 'Alzheimer's type dementia'*, Baltimore, MD: Health Professionals Press.

[99] For accounts of the Sonas sensory approach see:
Threadgold, M. (1995) 'Touching the soul through the senses', *Journal of Dementia Care*, vol 3, no 4, pp 18-20.

Ellis, J. and Thorn, T. (2000) 'Sensory stimulation: where do we go from here', *Journal of Dementia Care*, vol 8, no 1, pp 33-7.

[100] For an account of the RO approach see:
Holden, U. and Woods, R.T. (1995) *Positive approaches to dementia care*, 3rd edn, London: Churchill Livingstone.

[101] For an account of the Snoezelen approach see:
Dowling, Z., Baker, R., Wareing, L.A. and Assey, J. (1997) 'Lights, sounds and special effects', *Journal of Dementia Care*, vol 5, no 1, pp 16-18.

Ellis, J. and Thorn, T. (2000) 'Sensory stimulation: where do we go from here', *Journal of Dementia Care*, vol 8, no 1, pp 33-7.

[102] Perrin, T. (1997) 'Occupational need in severe dementia: a descriptive study', *Journal of Advanced Nursing*, no 25, pp 934-41.

[103] Perrin, T. (1995) 'A new pattern of life: re-assessing the role of occupation and activities', in T. Kitwood and S. Benson (eds) *The new culture of dementia care*, London: Hawker Publications, pp 66-9.

[104] For ideas for occupation and activities see:
Archibald, C. (1990) *Activities*, Stirling: Dementia Services Development Centre.

Archibald, C. (1993) *Activities II*, Stirling: Dementia Services Development Centre.

[105] Perrin, T. (1995) 'A new pattern of life: re-assessing the role of occupation and activities', in T. Kitwood and S. Benson (eds) *The new culture of dementia care*, London: Hawker Publications, pp 66-9.

[106] For example:
Perrin, T. and May, H. (1999) *Well-being in dementia: An occupational approach for therapists and carers*, London: Churchill Livingstone.

[107] Brooker, D. (2001) 'Enriching lives: evaluation of the ExtraCare activity challenge', *Journal of Dementia Care*, vol 9, no 3, pp 33-7.

Mealtimes and nutrition

[108] Chester, R. and Davis, S. (1997) *Appetite for life: Study of good practice around food and mealtimes in homes for older people*, London: Counsel and Care.

VOICES (1998) *Eating well for older people with dementia: A good practice guide for residential and nursing homes and others involved in caring for older people with dementia*, Expert Working Group on Eating Well for Older People with Dementia, Potters Bar: VOICES.

Physical and mental health

[109] Royal College of Physicians (2000) *The health and care of older people in care homes*, A report of a joint working party of the Royal College of Physicians, Royal College of Nursing and British Geriatrics Society, London: Royal College of Physicians.

[110] Moriarty, J. and Webb, S. (2000) *Part of their lives: Community care for older people with dementia*, Bristol: The Policy Press.

Medication

[111] Audit Commission (2000) *Forget me not: Mental health services for older people*, London: Audit Commission.

[112] DoH (2001d) *Medicines and older people: Implementing medicines-related aspects of the NSF for older people*, London: DoH.

[113] Levenson, R. (1998) *Drugs and dementia: A guide to good practice in the use of neuroleptic drugs in care homes for older people*, London: Age Concern.

Palliative care, death and dying

[114] Shemmings, Y. (1998) 'Death and dying in residential homes for older people', in R. Jack (ed) *Residential versus community care: The role of institutions in welfare provision*, Basingstoke: Macmillan, pp 154-65.

Counsel and Care (1995) *Last nights*, London: Counsel and Care.

[115] Cox, S., Gilhooly, M. and McLennan, J. (1997) *Dying and dementia*, Stirling: Dementia Services Development Centre.

Cox, S. (1994) 'Quality care for the dying person with dementia', *Journal of Dementia Care*, vol 4, no 4, pp 19-21.

Relatives

[116] Woods, B. (1999) *Partners in care: The interface between family care-givers and institutional care for people with Alzheimer's disease and related disorders*, Bangor: Dementia Services Development Centre, University of Wales.

[117] Moriarty, J. and Webb, S. (2000) *Part of their lives: Community care for older people with dementia*, Bristol: The Policy Press.

[118] Wright, F.D. (1998) *Continuing to care: The effect on spouses and children of an older person's admission to a care home*, York: York Publishing Services.

[119] Kitwood, T., Buckland, S. and Petre, T. (1995) *Brighter futures: A report on research into provision for persons with dementia in residential homes, nursing homes and sheltered housing*, Kidlington: Anchor Housing Association.

[120] DoH/Social Services Inspectorate (1993) *Standards for the residential care of elderly people with mental disorders*, Inspecting for Quality Series, London: HMSO.

[121] Alzheimer's Society (2000) *Alzheimer's Society response: Fit for the Future? National required standards for residential and nursing homes for older people*, London: Alzheimer's Society.

Community links

[122] Murphy, E., Lindesay, J. and Dean, R. (1994) *The Domus project: Long term care for older people with dementia*, London: Sainsbury Centre for Mental Health.

Kitwood, T., Buckland, S. and Petre, T. (1995) *Brighter futures: A report on research into provision for persons with dementia in residential homes, nursing homes and sheltered housing*, Kidlington: Anchor Housing Association.

[123] Cantley, C. (2001) 'Understanding people in organisations', in C. Cantley (ed) *A handbook of dementia care*, Buckingham: Open University Press.

Residents' money

[124] CPA (Centre for Policy on Ageing) (1996) *A better home life: A code of good practice for residential and nursing home care*, Advisory Group convened by Centre for Policy on Ageing, Chaired by Kina, Lady Avebury, London: CPA.

Office of Fair Trading (1998) *Older people as consumers in care homes: A report by the Office of Fair Trading*, OFT No 242, London: Office of Fair Trading.

Battison, T. (2000) *The everyday affairs: Training pack for use with care workers on basic legal and financial issues affecting older people*, London: Age Concern.

Jenkins, G. (1996) *Resident's money: A guide to good practice in care homes*, London: Age Concern.

Risk management

[125] Alaszewski, A., Harrison, L. and Manthorpe, J. (1998) *Risk, health and welfare: Policies, strategies and practice*, Buckingham: Open University Press.

[126] CPA (Centre for Policy on Ageing) (1996) *A better home life: A code of good practice for residential and nursing home care*, Advisory Group convened by Centre for Policy on Ageing, Chaired by Kina, Lady Avebury, London: CPA.

[127] Counsel and Care (1992b) *What if they hurt themselves: A discussion document on the uses and abuses of restraint in residential care homes and nursing homes*, London: Counsel and Care.

[128] Counsel and Care (1993) *The right to take risks*, London: Counsel and Care.

Pritchard, J. (1997) 'Vulnerable people taking risks: older people and residential care', in H. Kemshall and J. Pritchard (eds) *Good practice in risk assessment 2*, London: Jessica Kingsley Publishers.

[129] Counsel and Care (1992b) *What if they hurt themselves: A discussion document on the uses and abuses of restraint in residential care homes and nursing homes*, London: Counsel and Care.

Counsel and Care (1993) *The right to take risks*, London: Counsel and Care.

Alaszewski, A., Harrison, L. and Manthorpe, J. (1998) *Risk, health and welfare: Policies, strategies and practice*, Buckingham: Open University Press.

Gilloran, A., Robertson, A., McGlew, T. and McKee, K. (1995) 'Improving work satisfaction amongst nursing staff and quality of care for elderly patients with dementia: some policy implications', *Ageing and Society*, vol 15, no 3, pp 375-91.

Abuse

[130] Bright, L. (1999) 'Elder abuse in care and nursing settings: detection and prevention', in P. Slater and M. Eastman (eds) *Elder abuse: Critical issues in policy and practice*, London: Age Concern.

[131] Lawson, J. (1999) 'Developing a policy on abuse in residential and nursing homes', in J. Pritchard (ed) *Elder abuse work: Best practice in Britain and Canada*, London: Jessica Kingsley Publishers.

Griffin, J. (1999) 'Abuse in a safe environment', in J. Pritchard (ed) *Elder abuse work: Best practice in Britain and Canada*, London: Jessica Kingsley Publishers.

Home Office (2000) *No secrets: Guidance on developing and implementing multi-agency policies and procedures to protect vulnerable adults from abuse*, London: DoH.

[132] Royal College of Physicians (2000) *The health and care of older people in care homes*, A report of a joint working party of the Royal College of Physicians, Royal College of Nursing and British Geriatrics Society, London: Royal College of Physicians.

[133] Eastman, M. (1998) 'Why and when institutions do not work – *Sans everything* revisited', in R. Jack (ed) *Residential versus community care: The role of institutions in welfare provision*, Basingstoke: Macmillan.

Legal and ethical issues

[134] For general legal advice see, for example, chapters on residential and nursing homes in:
Mandelstam, M. (1999) *Community care practice and the law*, 2nd edn, London: Jessica Kingsley Publishers.

Clements, L. (2000) *Community care and the law*, 2nd edn, London: Legal Action Group.

For a discussion of law relating to people without mental capacity see:
Letts, P. (1999) 'The protection of people with mental incapacity', J. Pritchard (ed) *Elder abuse work: Best practice in Britain and Canada*, London: Jessica Kingsley Publishers.

Lord Chancellor's Department (1999) *Making decisions: The government's proposals for making decisions on behalf of mentally incapacitated adults*, Cm 4465, London: The Stationery Office.

For a discussion of ethical issues see, for example:
Stokes, G. (2001) 'Difficult decisions: what are a person's "best interests"?', *Journal of Dementia Care*, vol 9, no 3, pp 25-8.

Manthorpe, J. (2001) 'Ethical ideas and practice', in C. Cantley (ed) *A handbook of dementia care*, Buckingham: Open University Press.

Jaques, A. (1997) 'Ethical dilemmas in care and research for people with dementia', in S. Hunter (ed) *Dementia challenges and new directions*, Research Highlights in Social Work No 31, London: Jessica Kingsley Publishers, pp 24-41.

[135] Killeen, J. (1996) *Advocacy and dementia*, Edinburgh: Alzheimer Scotland – Action on Dementia.

[136] Marshall, M. (2001) 'Care settings and the care environment', in C. Cantley (ed) *A handbook of dementia care*, Buckingham: Open University Press.

Chapter 4: Staffing matters

[137] Netten, A. (1993) *A positive environment? Physical and social influences on people with senile dementia in residential care*, Aldershot/Canterbury: Ashgate/Personal Social Services Research Unit, University of Kent.

[138] Henwood, M. (2001) *Future imperfect: Report of the King's Fund Care & Support Inquiry*, London: King's Fund.

Staffing levels and skills

[139] Alzheimer's Society (2000) *Alzheimer's Society response: Fit for the Future? National required standards for residential and nursing homes for older people*, London: Alzheimer's Society.

[140] Marshall, M. (1998) 'Therapeutic buildings for people with dementia', in S. Judd, M. Marshall and P. Phippen (eds) *Design for dementia*, London: Hawker Publications, pp 11-14.

[141] Kitwood, T., Buckland, S. and Petre, T. (1995) *Brighter futures: A report on research into provision for persons with dementia in residential homes, nursing homes and sheltered housing*, Kidlington: Anchor Housing Association.

[142] Clarke, M. (1978) 'Getting through the work', in, R. Dingwall and J. McIntosh (eds) *Readings in sociology of nursing*, Edinburgh: Churchill Livingstone.

[143] Kitwood, T., Buckland, S. and Petre, T. (1995) *Brighter futures: A report on research into provision for persons with dementia in residential homes, nursing homes and sheltered housing*, Kidlington: Anchor Housing Association.

[144] Mountain, G. and Godfrey, M. (1995) *Respite care provision for older people with dementia: A review of the literature*, Leeds: Nuffield Institute for Health, University of Leeds.

Recruitment

[145] Herbert, G. (1997) 'What hat should we wear today? Recruiting and developing the ideal workforce for dementia care', in M. Marshall (ed) *State of the art in dementia care*, London: CPA, pp 111-15.

[146] Kitwood, T., Buckland, S. and Petre, T. (1995) *Brighter futures: A report on research into provision for persons with dementia in residential homes, nursing homes and sheltered housing*, Kidlington: Anchor Housing Association.

Herbert, G. (1997) 'What hat should we wear today? Recruiting and developing the ideal workforce for dementia care', in M. Marshall (ed) *State of the art in dementia care*, London: CPA, pp 111-15.

Packer, T. (1999) 'Attitudes towards dementia care: education and morale in health-care teams', in T. Adams and C. Clarke (eds) *Dementia care: Developing partnerships in practice*, London: Bailliere Tindall, pp 325-49.

[147] Perrin, T. (1997) 'Occupational need in severe dementia: a descriptive study', *Journal of Advanced Nursing*, no 25, pp 934-41.

[148] Clough, R. (2000) *The practice of residential work*, Basingstoke: Macmillan.

Herbert, G. (1997) 'What hat should we wear today? Recruiting and developing the ideal workforce for dementia care', in M. Marshall (ed) *State of the art in dementia care*, London: CPA, pp 111-15.

Work satisfaction

[149] Penna, S., Paylor, I. and Soothill, K. (1995) *Job satisfaction and dissatisfaction: A study of residential care work*, London: National Institute for Social Work.

[150] Penna, S., Paylor, I. and Soothill, K. (1995) *Job satisfaction and dissatisfaction: A study of residential care work*, London: National Institute for Social Work.

Kitwood, T., Buckland, S. and Petre, T. (1995) *Brighter futures: A report on research into provision for persons with dementia in residential homes, nursing homes and sheltered housing*, Kidlington: Anchor Housing Association.

Gilloran, A., Robertson, A., McGlew, T. and McKee, K. (1995) 'Improving work satisfaction amongst nursing staff and quality of care for elderly patients with dementia: some policy implications', *Ageing and Society*, vol 15, no 3, pp 375-91.

Moniz-Cook, E., Millington, D. and Silver, M. (1997) 'Residential care for older people: job satisfaction and psychological health in care staff', *Health and Social Care in the Community*, vol 5, no 2, pp 124-33.

Pay and conditions

[151] cf: Kitwood, T., Buckland, S. and Petre, T. (1995) *Brighter futures: A report on research into provision for persons with dementia in residential homes, nursing homes and sheltered housing*, Kidlington: Anchor Housing Association.

[152] Gilloran, A., Robertson, A., McGlew, T. and McKee, K. (1995) 'Improving work satisfaction amongst nursing staff and quality of care for elderly patients with dementia: some policy implications', *Ageing and Society*, vol 15, no 3, pp 375-91.

Staff development

[153] Ford, P. and Heath, H. (eds) (1996) *Nursing homes: Nursing values*, London: Royal College of Nursing.

Johnson, M.L., Cullen, L. and Patsios, D. (1999) *Managers in long-term care: Their quality and qualities*, Bristol/York: The Policy Press/Joseph Rowntree Foundation.

Alzheimer's Society (2000) *Alzheimer's Society response: Fit for the Future? National required standards for residential and nursing homes for older people*, London: Alzheimer's Society.

[154] DoH (2001a) *Care homes for older people: National minimum standards*, London: The Stationery Office.

[155] Archibald, C. (1997) *Specialist dementia units: A practice guide for staff*, Stirling: Dementia Services Development Centre.

Gilloran, A. and Downs, M. (1997) 'Issues of staffing and therapeutic care', in S. Hunter (ed) *Dementia challenges and new directions*, Research Highlights in Social Work No 31, London: Jessica Kingsley Publishers, pp 165-81.

Herbert, G. (1997) 'What hat should we wear today? Recruiting and developing the ideal workforce for dementia care', in M. Marshall (ed) *State of the art in dementia care*, London: CPA, pp 111-15.

Perrin, T. (1997) 'Occupational need in severe dementia: a descriptive study', *Journal of Advanced Nursing*, no 25, pp 934-41.

Proctor, R., Stratton-Powell, H., Tarrier, N. and Burns, A. (1998) 'The impact of training and support on stress among care staff in nursing and residential homes for the elderly', *Journal of Mental Health*, vol 7, no 1, pp 59-70.

[156] Kitwood, T. and Woods, B. (1996) *Training and development strategy for dementia care in residential settings*, Bradford: Bradford Dementia Group.

Alzheimer Scotland – Action on Dementia (2000) *Planning signposts for dementia care services*, Edinburgh: Alzheimer Scotland – Action on Dementia.

[157] Henwood, M. (2001) *Future imperfect: Report of the King's Fund Care & Support Inquiry*, London: King's Fund.

[158] Moniz-Cook, E., Millington, D. and Silver, M. (1997) 'Residential care for older people: job satisfaction and psychological health in care staff', *Health and Social Care in the Community*, vol 5, no 2, pp 124-33.

[159] Innes, A. (2000) *Training and development for dementia care workers*, Bradford Dementia Group Good Guides, London: Jessica Kingsley Publishers.

[160] Lintern, T., Woods, B. and Phair, L. (2000) 'Training is not enough to change care practice', *Journal of Dementia Care*, vol 8, no 2, pp 15-17.

Chapter 5: Design principles and processes

[161] Judd, S., Marshall, M. and Phippen, P. (eds) (1998) *Design for dementia*, London: Hawker Publications.

CAE (Centre for Accessible Environments) (1998) *The design of residential care and nursing homes for older people*, Health Facilities Note No 19, London: NHS Estates, DoH.

Brawley, E.C. (1997) *Designing for Alzheimer's disease: Strategies for creating better care environments*, New York, NY: John Wiley & Sons.

Dementia Services Development Centre (1997) *Design for dementia: Six conference papers*, Stirling: Dementia Services Development Centre.

Moos, R.H. and Lemke, S. (1996) *Evaluating residential facilities*, London: Sage Publications.

Stewart, S. and Page, A. (ed) (1999) *Just another disability: Making design dementia friendly*, Glasgow: Mackintosh School of Architecture, Glasgow School of Art.

Alzheimer Scotland – Action on Dementia (2000) *Planning signposts for dementia care services*, Edinburgh: Alzheimer Scotland – Action on Dementia.

DoH (2001a) *Care homes for older people: National minimum standards*, London: The Stationery Office.

Coles, R., Duncan, I., Kelly, M. and Wightman, A. (1992) *Signposts not barriers*, Stirling: Dementia Services Development Centre.

Marshall, M. (1997) *Dementia and technology*, London: Counsel and Care, sponsored by Methodist Homes for the Aged.

ASTRID (2000) *A guide to using technology within dementia care*, London: Hawker Publications.

Kelly, M. and Carr, J.S. (1995) *An evaluation of the design of specialist residential care units for people with dementia*, Stirling: Dementia Services Development Centre.

Wagland, J. and Peachment, G. (1995) *Chairs: Guidelines for the purchase of lounge, dining and occasional chairs for elderly long term residents*, Stirling: Dementia Services Development Centre.

[162] Judd, S., Marshall, M. and Phippen, P. (eds) (1998) *Design for dementia*, London: Hawker Publications.

[163] Alzheimer Scotland – Action on Dementia (2000) *Planning signposts for dementia care services*, Edinburgh: Alzheimer Scotland – Action on Dementia.

Chapter 7: Design consensus and debates

[164] DoH (2001a) *Care homes for older people: National minimum standards*, London: The Stationery Office.

[165] Coles, R., Duncan, I., Kelly, M. and Wightman, A. (1992) *Signposts not barriers*, Stirling: Dementia Services Development Centre.

[166] Marshall, M. (1997) *Dementia and technology*, London: Counsel and Care, sponsored by Methodist Homes for the Aged.

[167] ASTRID (2000) *A guide to using technology within dementia care*, London: Hawker Publications.

Chapter 8: Design recommendations

[168] Judd, S., Marshall, M. and Phippen, P. (eds) (1998) *Design for dementia*, London: Hawker Publications.

CAE (Centre for Accessible Environments) (1998) *The design of residential care and nursing homes for older people*, Health Facilities Note No 19, London: NHS Estates, DoH.

Stewart, S. and Page, A. (ed) (1999) *Just another disability: Making design dementia friendly*, Glasgow: Mackintosh School of Architecture, Glasgow School of Art.

DoH (2001a) *Care homes for older people: National minimum standards*, London: The Stationery Office.

Kelly, M. and Carr, J.S. (1995) *An evaluation of the design of specialist residential care units for people with dementia*, Stirling: Dementia Services Development Centre.

[169] Wagland, J. and Peachment, G. (1995) *Chairs: Guidelines for the purchase of lounge, dining and occasional chairs for elderly long term residents*, Stirling: Dementia Services Development Centre.

Appendix: Comparison of various aspects of care homes visited

	Home A	Home B	Home C	Home D	Home E	Home F	Suggestions for inclusion in in design brief and specification*
Opened	1993	1997	1996	1993	1996	1996	
Category	Nursing	Residential	Residential	Dual registered	Residential	Nursing	
Organisation	Charity	Charity	Not for profit	HA	Not for profit	Charity	
Setting	Urban	Suburban	Suburban	Suburban	Suburban	Edge of town	
Costs (at time of construction)							
Build cost: including fixed equipment	£895,500	£1,868,000	£1,778,000 inc. day centre D&B all inclusive	£1,299,600	£1,354,700	£1,790,000 inc. day centre	
	D&B			D&B	D&B	D&B	
Build cost per place†	£24,800	£51,800	£29,600	£54,150	£18,800	£68,800	
Overall: excluding land	£1,145,366	£2,280,137	£1,778,000	£1,771,325	£1,718,230	£2,108,800	
Design factors							
Design concept	Group living	Group living	Group living	Group living	Large group	Group living	Group living
Number of floors	2	1 + part basement	2	2	1	2+part 2nd floor	Site and budget
Number of residents	36	36	60	24	72	26	40-60
Group size	9	12	15	8	24	3/7/8/8	8-15
					Domestic style		
General							
Site constraints	Size and shape	Contours	None – rebuild	Size and shape	Shallow	Tight site	
Design brief available	Yes	Yes – repeat	Standard brief	Dev with arch	Dev with arch	Yes	Site and budget
Wheelchair accessible	Yes	Yes	Yes	Yes	Yes	Yes	Yes
Staff:resident ratio	1:4.5 (plus % senior)	1:4	1:5	1:4	1:8	1:4 + % senior	
Floor area (m²)							
Gross	1,584	2,029	2,332	1,192	2,458	1,620 exc. daycentre	
Gross per resident	44	56	38.9	49.7	34.1	62.3	45-50
Day space per resident	6.5	9.6	5.5 + daycentre	10.3	4.2	c. 7 + daycentre	6+

Appendix: contd.../

	Home A	Home B	Home C	Home D	Home E	Home F	Suggestions for inclusion in in design brief and specification*
Group wing							
Group size	9	12	15	8	24	3/7/8/8	8–15
Resident rooms							
Resident room: gross	16.9	16.9	15.1/15.8	16	13.3	18	17 minimum
Net usable space (m²)	10.9	11.6	12.2	10.5	10.8	11.8	12 minimum
Shape of main space	3.4 x 3.2	3.4 x 3.4	3.2 x 3.8	3.6 x 2.9	3 x 3.6	3.7 x 3.0	
Fitted wardrobe	No	No	No	Yes – too small	No	No	Yes
Telephone point	For payphone	Yes	Yes	Use mobile	Yes	Yes + fax	Yes
Television aerial socket	Yes	Yes	Yes	Yes	Yes	Yes	Yes
En suite area (m²)	4	3	2.68/3.27	4	1.8 ave	3.4	4 minimum
Shower	Yes	No	No	In 4 en suites	No	No	Yes
Door	Opens both ways	Opens both ways	Opens outwards	Opens outwards	1.5 doors outwards	Opens outwards	Opens both ways
Day space							
Total floor area (m²)	58.8	71	n/a	41	n/a	n/a	
Per resident	6.53	5.92	n/a	5.13	n/a	n/a	
Sitting room or area	32.8	38.5	35	24.6	3 x 20.2 = 60.6	30	
Per resident	3.64	3.21	2.33	3.1	2.53	3.75	
Dining room or area	26	22	33	12.6	40	20	
Per resident	2.9	1.83	2.2	1.6	1.67	2.5	
Kitchenette/facilities	5.9	10.5	8	3.8	13.8 servery	3.8	Yes – in dining area
Access to grounds	Yes	Yes	Yes	Yes	To court from dining	Yes	Yes
Other sitting areas	None	4.2 at end corridor	3 at end corridor	Corridor recesses	None	Entrance and first floor	Desirable

Appendix: contd.../

	Home A	Home B	Home C	Home D	Home E	Home F	Suggestions for inclusion in in design brief and specification*
Assisted bathroom							
Ratio per resident	1:9	1:6	1:15	1:8	(2) 1:12	1:8	As regulations
Floor area (m²)	9	11.55	12	15	10.4	10	11
Assisted bath	Yes	Yes	Yes	Yes	Yes	Yes	Yes
Shower	No	Yes	No	Upper floor only	No	Yes	Yes
WC	Yes	Yes	Yes	Yes	Yes	Yes	Yes
Wash hand basin	Yes	Yes	Yes	Yes	Yes	Yes	Yes
Assisted shower room							
Ratio per resident	n/a	n/a	1:15	n/a	(1) 1:24	n/a	
Floor area	n/a	n/a	9	n/a	6.3	n/a	
Shower	n/a	n/a	Yes	n/a	Yes	n/a	
WC	n/a	n/a	Yes	n/a	Yes	n/a	
Wash hand basin	n/a	n/a	Yes	n/a	Yes	n/a	
Assisted WC							
Floor area (m²)	4	4.27	4	2.8	2 x 3.0	3.2	4
Clean linen store							
Floor area (m²)	3	8.75	1.6	2.4	2 x 1.45	3.2 Gf and 2.25 1st fl	6
Utility/sluice room							
Floor area (m²)	None	7.3	3	None	4	8.3 Gfl and 3.2 1st fl	4-6
Sluice/bedpan washer	None	Yes	Yes	Yes – in laundry	Yes	Yes	Yes
Other	None	Sink and worktop	None	None	None	Well equipped	
Cleaner's facility							
Floor area (m²)	1.25	1.54	0.6	2.4	1.5	3.2 Gfl and 1.25 1st fl	1.5 minimum
Equipment/materials	In store	In store	In store	In store	In store	In store	
Deep sink	No	Yes	No	Yes	Yes	Yes	Yes

Appendix: contd.../

	Home A	Home B	Home C	Home D	Home E	Home F	Suggestions for inclusion in in design brief and specification*
General storage							
Area	None	50	None	None	Limited	3.5 Gfl and 6.4 1st fl	0.75m²/res.
Location	n/a	In roof space	n/a	n/a	Various	Centrally	Various
Corridors							
Minimum width (m)	1.4	1.5	1.6	1.4	1.55	1.5 min	1.5 minimum
Varied width	Yes	Yes	Yes	Yes	No	Yes	Yes
Maximum length (m)	13	14.7	22	19	19	23.8	
Natural light	Borrowed	End and borrowed	At end only	End and borrowed	At ends	Borrowed	Preferable
Doors							
Varied colours	Bold on res door	Pastel on res door	No	No	Yes	No – wood	Vary colours
Special identification	None	Photos or pictures	Name plates	None	Small panel + no.	A4 frame with no.	A4 panel minimum
Main home facilities							
Main lounge							
Area (m²)	None	120 central foyer	None	55	None	None	If specified
Access to grounds	n/a	Yes	n/a	Yes	n/a	n/a	Yes
Space for all residents	No	Yes	With day centre	Yes	No	Can use day centre	Desirable
Entrance lobby							
Area (m²)	8	12.3	7	5	5.8	None	8
Door-entry system	Yes	Yes	No	No	Yes	n/a	Yes
Entrance/reception							
Area (m²)	c. 17	None	69 with rec desk	40 with rec desk	12 with desk	54 with desk	To suit need
Door-entry system	Yes	Yes	Yes	Yes	Yes	Yes	Yes
Separate staff entrance	No	Yes	No	Yes	Yes	No	Yes
Disabled WC							
Area (m²)	4 – one per floor	3.8/3.4	3	3.2	3.5	2 x 3.6 Gfl	3.5 minimum

Appendix: contd.../

'Put yourself in my place'

	Home A	Home B	Home C	Home D	Home E	Home F	Suggestions for inclusion in in design brief and specification*
Visitor WC	Yes	Yes	Yes	No	Use of disabled WC	Use of disabled WC	Yes
Other day space							
1) Area (m²)	14	None	46	15	Recesses	10	c. 20
use	Snoezelen – 1st fl	n/a	Sun lounge	Hobbies	Overlook courts	Chapel/quiet – gr fl	Quiet room
2) Area (m²)	None	None	9.4	15	None	10	
use	n/a	n/a	Smoking – 1st fl	Conservatory	n/a	Quiet – 1st fl	
Pay 'phone	Mobile unit	Staff/visitors	No	No – use cordless	No – use cordless	No – use cordless	
Ancillary accommodation							
Guest room – double							
Area (m²)	None	15.2	15.5	Use interview room	None	None	No
Location	n/a	Admin wing	res room if available	See above	n/a	n/a	n/a
Guest room – single (or staff sleep over)							
Area (m²)	n/a	11.4	n/a	11	n/a	16	No
Location	n/a	Admin wing	n/a	n/a	n/a	2nd floor	n/a
Home manager's office							
Area (m²)	None – uses Snoezelen	18.25	17	11	10	11.5 + store	12–15
Location	None	Off central foyer	First floor	Behind ent foyer	Entrance	Adj gen office	Near entrance
General office							
Area (m²)	9	13.3	17	None	8	20	15
Location	Near entrance	Admin wing	Near entrance	Share manager's	Near entrance	Near entrance	Near entrance
Counsel/meeting room							
Area (m²)	None	16.8	17	9.4	15	29.4	15 – if provided
Location	n/a	Admin wing	First floor	Admin wing	Near entrance	End ground floor	Admin area

Appendix

Appendix: contd.../

	Home A	Home B	Home C	Home D	Home E	Home F	Suggestions for inclusion in in design brief and specification*
Handover/training room							
Area (m²)	Use staff rest room	18.4	17	Use staff rest room	None	16.5	15 – if provided
Location	First floor	Admin wing	Next gen off	Admin wing	n/a	Services wing	Admin area
Staff rest room							
1) area (m²)	22.36	24.75	18.7 non-smoking	12.1	10.6 non-smoking	12.2 + kitchen	Related to number
location	First floor	Admin wing	First floor	Admin wing	Near entrance	First-floor cottage	
2) area (m²)	None	None	17 smoking	None	7.8 smoking	None	
location	n/a	n/a	First floor	n/a	Near entrance	n/a	
Changing: female	5	20.4	18.9	7.2 with lockers	11	22.7	15 minimum
Changing: male	3.25	9.5	Unisex!	5.9 with sh and WC	12	10.8	10 minimum
Treatment							
Area (m²)				8.1	11.5	To requirements	
Location					Near entrance	Services wing	
Nurse station							
Area (m²)	1.0 – open				4.7	3.7 each floor	To requirements
Location	Central each wing				One each wing	Centrally	
Care manager's office							
Area (m²)					8.6		Reflects size of home
Location					Near entrance		
Support facilities							
Hairdressing salon							
Area (m²)	None	15	12	Comb hobbies	7	16	12
Location	Use adj home	Off central foyer	First floor	Off ent foyer	Off central walkway	Services wing	Shared use?
Frequency of service	Weekly	Weekly	Weekly	Weekly	3 x per week	?	To suit demand

Appendix: contd.../

	Home A	Home B	Home C	Home D	Home E	Home F	Suggestions for inclusion in in design brief and specification*
'Shop'							
Location	None	Space available	Trolley	None	Off central walkway	None	
Opening times	n/a	n/a	2 hours Wed	n/a	Not used (storage)	n/a	
Main kitchen							
Area (m²)	35 + stores	48 + stores	57 + stores	27.8 + stores	37 + stores	35 + trolley park	35-40
Area per resident (m²)	0.97	1.33	0.95	1.15	0.51	1.34	>1
Cooking regime	On site	On site	On site	On site	On site	On site	To suit
Stores area (m²)	6.25	28	8	2.2	21.6	16.7	<16
Stores number	1	3	2	3	3	3	3
Location	Near main ent	End admin wing	Serv wing – front	Behind lounge	Adj kitchen/entrance	End services wing	To suit layout
Staffing	Chef +	Chef +	Chef +	Chef +	Chef +	Chef +	
Main laundry							
Area – internal (m²)	18.5	35.8	37	16	35	20	25-35
Location	GrFl front	End admin wing	GrFl front	Rear centre	Rear att. bungalow	Services wing	To suit layout
Staffing	Regular staff	Part time plus rota	Varied	Dedicated staff	Yes	Dedicated + night	Dedicated
Area – external drying (m²)	None	20	None	22	external drying	None	Small area desirable
Utility/sluice							
Area (m²)	8/11.34	On group wing	Sluice on each wing	Sluice in laundry	Sluice on each wing	Each floor	See Group area
Sluice/bedpan washer	Yes	See above	See above	See above	Yes	See above	As above
Other	Access to laundry	n/a	n/a	n/a	n/a	n/a	n/a
Location	See above	See above	see above	See above	Corner wing	Each floor	
Clean linen							
Area (m²)	See below	n/a	See below	3.7	On wings	See above	See Group area
Location	On group wing	On group wing	In laundry	In central core	Off corridors	See above	

Appendix: contd.../

	Home A	Home B	Home C	Home D	Home E	Home F	Suggestions for inclusion in in design brief and specification*
Separate staff toilet	Yes	Yes	Yes	Yes	Yes	Yes	Yes
Pharmacy store							
Area (m²)	0.75	Secure trolley	12	8.1	Treatment room	2.7	3 to 5
Location	Central on wing	Various	1st fl + units/wing	Admin wing	Near entrance	Off manager's office	Near manager
Storage							
Total area (m²)	None	19.3	65	14	5	20 gr floor; 6.6 1st and 10 2nd floor	15
Location	No gen storage	Various	Mainly first floor	Ground floor	Near laundry		To suit layout
Wheelchair storage							
Area (m²)	3.6	None	None	Used as gen store	5.4	None	Yes
Plant room							
Area (m²)	4.2	43.75	19	12.8	13.8	48 in roof space	To suit layout
Workshop							
Area (m²)	None	14.25	None	Shed in grounds	None	22 inc store	16
Garden store							
Area (m²)	None	16	Shed provided	See above	None	1.25	Included in above
Refuse							
Internal – area (m²)	None allocated	16	None	None	None	5.7	
Internal – location	n/a	Lower floor	n/a	n/a	n/a	Near kitchen	
External – area (m²)	10.5	Collection area only	c. 100 in yard	8	Not defined	None	External only
External – location	Near access	See above	Adj to kitchen	Outside admin	Near laundry and kitchen	n/a	
Day care centre							
Capacity	n/a	n/a	10	n/a	n/a	10	To specification
Area (m²)	n/a	n/a	63	n/a	n/a	71.5	Aas above
Location	n/a	n/a	Near entrance	n/a	n/a	Adj entrance	

Appendix: contd.../

	Home A	Home B	Home C	Home D	Home E	Home F	Suggestions for inclusion in in design brief and specification*
Stairs							
Minimum width (m)	1	1.1	1	1	n/a	1.1	1.1
Access – secure	Yes	Yes	No	No – soon	n/a	No	Yes
Lift							
Capacity	6 person	8 person	8 person	8 person	n/a	2 x 8 person	8 person
Special features	None	Only for deliveries	Two sets of doors	Long and narrow	n/a	Standard	As required
Heating							
Type	Gas – wet – LST rads	Gas – wet – LST rads	Gas – wet – LST rads	Underfl and ceiling	Gas – wet – LST rads	Low pressure wet	
Furniture in contract	No	No	Yes	No	No	No	
Gardens							
Continuous paths	Yes	Yes	Yes	Yes	No	Yes	Yes
Special features							
Seating	Yes	Yes	Yes with arbours	Yes	In courts	Yes	Yes
Greenhouse	Shed	Yes	Yes	Yes	No	No	Space for future
Other 1	Two main gardens	Garden/wing	Ornamental pond	3 col schemes	Inner courtyards	Arbor walk	Specialist design
Other 2	Grassed areas	Grassed areas	Grassed areas	Private areas	Sloping grass only	Level grass area	
Other 3	Selective planting	Select planting	Selective planting	Selective planting		Selective planting	
Other 4	Paved terraces	Terrace/wing	Paved terraces	Paved terraces		Paved terrace	
Other 5	Car in garden	Vegetable garden	Raised beds	Raised beds		Raised beds	
Other 6	Summer house		Aviary		Gazebo	Circular path	
Other 7			Footpath lighting			Covered terrace	
Maintenance	Contract	On site	Contract	20 hours/wk	On site and contractor	Company team	

Appendix

Notes:
* The final column contains suggestions for inclusion in a design brief and specification based on our findings.
† The variation in capital cost per resident place results from a combination of factors:
- the degree of simplicity versus complexity in the design
- the specification of materials, equipment and fittings
- the repetition in elements of design, for example the three identical bungalows in Home E
- the gross floor area per resident, for example compare Homes E and F
- the incorporation of a day centre
- regional and time differences in building cost rates.

Key

arch	architect
adj	adjacent
D&B	Design and Build
ent	entrance
1st fl	first floor
gen	general
Gfl	ground floor
inc	including
ha	housing association
off	office
rec	reception
res	resident
sh	shower
LST rads	low surface temperature radiators
underfl	underfloor heating
Wed	Wednesday
serv	services